WOMEN AND HEALTH

Cultural and Social Perspectives

Reproductive HEALTH, Reproductive RIGHTS

REFORMERS AND THE POLITICS OF MATERNAL WELFARE, 1917–1940

Robyn L. Rosen

 THE OHIO STATE UNIVERSITY PRESS
Columbus

Library of Congress Cataloging-in-Publication Data

Rosen, Robyn L.
    Reproductive health, reproductive rights : reformers and the politics of
maternal welfare, 1917–1940 / Robyn L. Rosen.
        p. cm. — (Women and health)
Includes bibliographical references and index.
        ISBN 0-8142-0920-3 (alk. paper) — ISBN 0-8142-9009-4 (CD-ROM)

1. Maternal and infant welfare—United States—History—20th century.
2. Maternal health services—United States—History—20th century. 3. Reproductive
health—United States—History—20th century. 4. Birth control—United States—
History—20th century. 5. Women's rights—United States—History—20th century.
6. Women social reformers—United States—Biography. I. Title. II. Women & health
(Columbus, Ohio)
    HV699.R66 2003
    362.83—dc21
                            2002155437

Jacket design by Melissa Ryan.
Type set in Adobe Caslon.
Printed by Thomson-Shore, Inc.

The paper used in this publication meets the minimum requirements of the American
National Standard for Information Sciences—Permanence of Paper for Printed Library
Materials. ANSI Z39.48-1992.

9 8 7 6 5 4 3 2 1

Contents

Series Editors' Preface

Robyn Rosen's book *Reproductive Health, Reproductive Rights: Reformers and the Politics of Maternal Welfare, 1917–1940* uses a biographical approach to present critical issues in the history of women's reproductive health and rights. Rather than focusing on Margaret Sanger, the extremely influential national leader of the birth control movement, Rosen brings to the forefront four other vital leaders whose contributions have not received the attention they deserve. Elizabeth Lowell Putnam, Ethel Sturges Dummer, Mary Ware Dennett, and Blanche Ames were all well-known contemporaries of Sanger. Though all were active in the areas of women's health and reproductive rights, each had a unique approach to the reproductive issues women faced. Rosen's nuanced biographies pay particular attention to the relations among her subjects. She weighs the various and changing views of each of these activists and compares their approaches—assessing their sometimes unified and sometimes divided interpretations of women's needs. Her book demonstrates the complicated politics of the era while making clear that reproductive health and access to birth control was a major historical subject.

We are pleased to include *Reproductive Health, Reproductive Rights* in our series. We believe that its critical historical insights have much to offer and that these women can enhance our understanding of the complexities of reproductive politics that are present today in the twenty-first century.

— RIMA D. APPLE AND JANET GOLDEN, SERIES EDITORS

Acknowledgments

Throughout the research, writing, and revision of this book I have incurred many debts, which I am pleased to have the opportunity to acknowledge.

The original research for this book was funded in great part by the Department of History at Binghamton University. Additional support was received from the Schlesinger Library and the Rockefeller Archives. I would like to thank the archivists at the Sophia Smith Collection, the Schlesinger Library, the Rockefeller Archives, and the National Archives for their valuable assistance. Indiana University Press and Blackwell Publishers have granted me permission to reprint portions of this material from the following sources: Sonya Michel and Robyn Rosen, "The Paradox of Maternalism: Elizabeth Lowell Putnam and the American Welfare State," *Gender and History* (autumn 1992): 364–85; and Robyn Rosen, "Federal Expansion, Fertility Control, and Physicians in the U.S.: The Politics of Maternal Welfare in the Interwar Years," *Journal of Women's History* 10, no. 3 (autumn 1998): 53–73.

Over the years, several scholars have read the manuscript in part or in its entirety (some several times over) and generously offered to share their knowledge of women's history. These include: Katherine Kish Sklar, Sonya Michel, Molly Ladd-Taylor, Lynne Curry, Lee Ann Wheeler, and Patricia West. Their insights have all made the book a better one. Chapter 1 owes a special debt to Sonya Michel, whose gracious offer to collaborate during the earliest stages of my research helped me on my way. Patricia West has generously and lovingly provided me with intellectual and emotional support at crucial moments during this long process that has kept me from losing my way several times.

Acquisitions Editor, Heather Lee Miller, has been wonderfully professional and supportive during the process of turning this manuscript into a book and I thank her for her time and her faith in this project. Copyediting Coordinator Karie Kirkpatrick has likewise been a great help and a pleasure to work with.

I am lucky enough to have colleagues at Marist College who share a dedication to teaching and scholarship and make my job rewarding and fun. Many thanks to my colleagues, past and present, in the School of Liberal Arts and particularly the Department of History for their professionalism, support, and friendship. A special thanks to Thom Wermuth for his professional guidance and friendship over the years.

I have been sustained through the writing of this book by the love of family and friends. Thanks to Diane and Shari for your lifetime of love and support and for showing me what strong, happy women can do with their lives. Thanks to Alex and Jane for awaiting this book's publication with so much loving anticipation, and for being such wonderful grandparents to my boys. Thanks to the Higuera family for becoming my family, and especially to Laraine for a million kindnesses over the years. For providing great meals, parties, vacations, shopping trips, a best friend for Nate, and for always coming early and staying late, thanks to Betsy and Shawn. For their special kind of Minnesotan hospitality and friendship over the years, thanks to Richard and Leigh. For her love of women's history, and her energy and optimism in the face of a daunting balancing act, thanks to Sally Dwyer-McNulty. For their love and faith in me over all these years, many thanks to my old and dear friends Meredith, Sully, Jill, Ronni, Thea, and Anke. For enriching my life in Berkshire County through their friendship, thanks to Deborah and Pam. For much-needed nights out each month, lots of laughs, conversation, and good food, thanks to my book group. For caring for my children over the years so I could teach, write, and spend a few minutes by myself, thanks to Leslie and Sue.

In the end, this book is dedicated to my guys:

To Vinnie, for being a wonderful partner who makes every accomplishment possible and for hanging in, remembering to laugh, and always loving us in spite of the craziness.

To Nate, whose entire life so far has coincided with writing of this book, for turning me into a mother, for surpassing so many of my expectations of how a child of mine might turn out, for your intensity, your sense of style, and for showing the little boys the way.

To Louis, for your positively limitless supply of affection, and your curiosity about this great big world.

To Sam, for giving me the joy of mothering just one last chubby, happy baby.

Introduction

Shortly after the United States entered World War I, philanthropist Ethel Sturges Dummer wrote to her friend Katharine Anthony expressing the hope that the war would encourage a scientific reexamination of "the whole problem of motherhood and the relation of the child to the state."[1] Dummer's sentiments in 1917 point to a critical moment when traditional nineteenth-century concern for the welfare of women and children converged with new public health standards and notions of modern motherhood.[2] Significantly, this period also shifted away from Victorian sensibilities about family limitation and sexuality. Thus, women's reproductive lives received unprecedented public attention as women's sexual and maternal identity destabilized in the early twentieth century.[3] This book explores the highly charged politics of reproduction that emerged in this era of transitions. It explores how, between 1910 and 1939, the movement for women's reproductive rights was estranged from the movement for women's reproductive health.

To analyze this trajectory of alienation, this book focuses on the political careers of four reformers: Elizabeth Lowell Putnam (1862–1935), Ethel Sturges Dummer (1866–1954), Mary Dennett (1872–1947), and Blanche Ames (1878–1969). All engaged in political activism on behalf of mothers during the Progressive Era and into the interwar years, reflecting diverse goals, temperaments, and strategies. Together, their careers offer a lens through which to discern the political circumstances that shaped movements for maternal justice, rights, and health. This lens allows us to examine the constellation of forces that contended to advance or thwart the firm establishment of women's reproductive rights and health care within the domains of policy and culture in the transitional decades of the early twentieth century.

The separate histories of the movements for reproductive health and reproductive rights have been well documented by other scholars. This book highlights points of connection and disagreement. Rarely have accounts of women's activism acknowledged the connections between efforts to legalize contraception and concurrent efforts to improve maternal and infant health.[4]

The infant and maternal welfare movement, always the more respectable and mainstream of the two, has its origins in public health reform of the late nineteenth century. Infant mortality was one of the first problems tackled by public health reformers, as they considered it an accurate measure of community health standards.[5] When women began to join and even lead the fight against infant mortality, the movement already enjoyed a status that made it more than a mother's issue. By the early twentieth century it had deep roots in the burgeoning public health bureaucracies throughout the country. Local, state, and municipal governments were the first to develop, fund, and administer programs designed to protect the health of mothers and children. The passage of mothers' pensions, food and milk regulation, and housing and sanitary reforms all illustrate the commitment of state resources.

The federal government joined this movement with the 1909 White House Conference on the Care of Dependent Children. According to historian Kristen Lindenmeyer, the conference reflected a shift from nineteenth-century "child saving" toward "twentieth century–style child welfare techniques emphasizing prevention, government regulation, [and] aid to families so that children might stay within their own homes."[6] The idea of creating a federal bureau dedicated to children was first seriously considered at the 1909 White House Conference.

Three years later, the U.S. Children's Bureau (CB) was established in the Department of Labor to "investigate and report upon all matters pertaining to the welfare of children and child life."[7] With the creation of the CB, women reformers, settlement house workers, and social scientists entered the "mostly male empire of policymaking."[8] The CB, created prior to women's enfranchisement but at the height of women's civic and political power, gave women reformers a powerful base from which to assert their vision. This vision centered around research into and support for poor, disabled, and disadvantaged children. With the passage of the Sheppard-Towner Maternity and Infancy Protection Act in 1921, the CB initiated, designed, and administered a nationally coordinated effort to tackle infant mortality and eventually maternal mortality. Both Ethel Dummer and Elizabeth Putnam involved themselves in the creation and early activities of the CB.

On the one hand, the origins of the birth control movement can also be found in nineteenth-century public health concerns. Neo-Malthusians, who argued that population growth led to poverty and suffering, were among the first to promote the use of artificial contraception to solve these social problems. On the other hand, the birth control movement also boasted a more radical heritage. Free love radicals, utopian socialists, feminists, and anarchists counted themselves among the first advocates of birth control. Unlike reproductive health campaigns that promised to improve family health and welfare, these latter birth control reformers posed and/or were interpreted as posing overt challenges to the institutions of marriage, monogamy, the nuclear family, and the dominant paradigms regarding female sexuality and mothering. To guard against these threats, Congress passed federal obscenity laws in 1873 that included birth control in their definition of obscenity. By the early twentieth century anxiety over such things as free love, pornography, prostitution, perversion, and "white slavery" manifested in a repressive, if often arbitrarily enforced, legal code. Thus, while maternal and infant welfare began to attract federal attention in the form of investigation and financial appropriation, birth control attracted government censorship and prohibition in the same decades.

Faced with repression and opposition, early-twentieth-century birth control reformers pioneered a variety of creative tactics to disassociate their cause from its checkered past. In an attempt to move into mainstream American culture, reformers appropriated discourses that would attract rather than repel most Americans. In the place of radical critiques of American society and culture, birth controllers now offered sentimental stories about mothers and babies, patriotic sentiments about the vigor of American citizens, rational arguments for scientific and medical progress, and, finally, eugenic ideas that advocated a healthier and usually less diverse society. By the time married people could legally obtain birth control materials under limited circumstances in the 1930s, the cause had been thoroughly sanitized by savvy and pragmatic reformers. Dennett and Ames provided significant leadership among these innovative birth control reformers.

Despite their distinct origins and encounters with public policy, by the interwar years the movements also shared some fundamental tenets. In the Progressive Era, liberal thinkers began to articulate a vision of an ever-improving society, advocating conscious intervention to correct or compensate for the problems wrought by industrial excess. Reproductive reform campaigns reflected this determination to challenge fate, to create options where none had seemed to exist, and to develop strategies to improve circumstances. The "discovery" of excessively high infant mortality rates illustrated this new way of thinking about the world. Mortality rates can only be considered excessive if people believe that these deaths could and should be prevented. Historian Richard Meckel makes this point when he writes that infant welfare reformers "helped transform a demographic condition into a social problem."[9] Similarly, research into population growth and public health grew out of new confidence in the possibility of subverting what had heretofore been considered natural phenomena. Movements to challenge the inevitability of infant death, maternal death, unchecked childbearing, and limitations placed on women's personal fulfillment flourished within this cultural milieu. Thus, the roots of the reproductive health and rights movements can be found in similar orientations toward the relation between fate and progress, inevitability and intervention.

In addition to common goals and orientations, the movements for reproductive health and reproductive rights were shaped by many of the same political and historical circumstances. Both gained greater acceptance on the heels of wartime concerns over the health of U.S. soldiers and citizens, high mortality rates, sexually transmitted diseases, and epidemics; both developed ambivalent relations with the organized medical community that ultimately shaped their respective fates; both were caught up in debates about the welfare state, eugenics, the quality of women's lives, and the fate of the American family.

Three main threads of analysis run through this study. First, political diversity among white middle- and upper-class female reformers in the interwar years reveals itself through comparative examination of their work in the birth control and maternal and infant welfare movements. While many female reformers shared concern over the health and welfare of mothers and babies, political considerations and orientations led women reformers in distinct and sometimes competing directions. Examining the constellation of political causes related to reproduction that surrounded, attracted, and repelled the women in this study, this book offers a novel perspective on women's political opportunities and choices in the early twentieth century.

Second, each movement, that for infant and maternal health on the one hand, and birth control on the other, can be understood more fully by acknowledging the historical presence of the other. By considering each movement's variable fortunes and failures in the context of the other, we see more clearly the political circumstances that shaped both movements. Specifically, this study examines and compares the varied impacts of maternalist and feminist rhetoric, political alliances, and legislative strategies on reproductive rights and reproductive health activism.

Third, this study argues that our understanding of the reproductive health mainstream—the Children's Bureau—and the reproductive rights mainstream—Margaret Sanger and the "Sangerists"—can be enhanced through an examination of their relations with associates and rivals from within the reproductive reform arena. While Putnam, Dummer, Dennett, and Ames all provided leadership in reproductive reform circles, they initiated breaks with and found themselves marginalized by the mainstream for ideological and tactical reasons that I will explore. Identifying and analyzing the factors that contributed to these tensions offers a new perspective on recognized leaders. This study reassesses the scope of their leadership, the wisdom of their vision, and their location along the political spectrum.

The first part of this book focuses on two reformers who worked with and against the CB to improve the lives of mothers and children. Elizabeth Lowell Putnam and Ethel Sturges Dummer, the wealthiest women in this study, were dedicated reformers and philanthropists. While both provided crucial aid to the CB in its early years—promoting its activities to women's groups and politicians, as well as providing advice and financial assistance—ideological and political differences would undermine relations with the CB by the end of their careers. Putnam would become an enemy of the CB by the 1920s, embracing fiscal conservatism and joining the ranks of red-baiting patriots. Dummer, on the other hand, simply lost faith in the CB's ability to stand up for women's interests and moved on to other causes. Putnam and Dummer's political careers, as they intersected and clashed with policy makers in the CB, help to expose the CB's achievements and innovations, as well as its compromises and flaws.

Chapter 1 traces the dramatic political career of Elizabeth Lowell Putnam. Putnam dedicated her life to lowering infant and maternal mortality rates first though milk reform and then through pioneering work in prenatal care. Unlike the overwhelming majority of female welfare reformers in the interwar years, Putnam came of age politically as an antisuffragist. A wealthy Boston Brahmin, Putnam held traditional views on the proper roles of both women and the federal government. Even as she helped form and shape the agenda of the maternal and infant welfare movement, she became an outspoken critic of federal expansion or regulation in this arena. Although neither a suffragist nor a feminist, Putnam can be called a "maternalist," meaning she utilized nineteenth-century notions of motherhood to legitimate women's civic activism on behalf of women and children.[10] A comparison of Putnam's pre- and postwar activities highlights the diminishing effectiveness of maternalist ideology as a unifying force among U.S. female reformers.

Putnam's story reveals that major fault lines among women reformers tended to rest on attitudes toward the state and conventional left-to-right political affiliations, rather than on different levels of commitment to maternal and infant health. Indeed, Putnam was as dedicated to saving the lives of mothers and infants as the women in the CB, but her political orientation yielded a different path: away from the plight of the poor and from federally sponsored social welfare programs.[11] This is a path that historians of women are less familiar with, but one that nevertheless reveals the varieties of forms that reproductive reform could take in the interwar years. Her political career defies conventional categorization and thus complicates our understanding of women's political culture. Her dedication to maternal and infant welfare veered off the path taken by most maternalists, as she combined some early tendencies—an orientation towards the middle class rather than the poor, and a faith in medical rather than holistic solutions to the problems of mothers and infants—with a political program of small government articulated by right-wing groups that began to emerge in the 1920s. Putnam, therefore, helps us to understand both the ways in which maternalism could facilitate alliances, and its limitations as an organizing principle.

Chapter 2 presents the contrasting career of philanthropist and reformer Ethel Sturges Dummer. It traces the development of Dummer's feminist politics and her important role as a philanthropist in the arena of maternal welfare and sexual reform. Although she is the least politically active figure in this study, Dummer involved herself in some of the most controversial reform campaigns that comprised reproductive reform, attempting to establish equal rights for unwed mothers and their children, an adequate system of financial support for all mothers, and an end to the sexual double standard.[12] While Dummer worked with the highest-ranking staff of the CB to enact legislation, educate the public, and improve maternal and infant welfare services, her positions were shaped by a different set of sensibilities and goals. Foremost among these differences was Dummer's conviction that motherhood was unnecessarily problematic due to women's subordinate social position. Dummer's career highlights the distinctions between feminist and maternalist approaches to maternal welfare. For the CB, problems arose when mothers were unable to fulfill their responsibilities to their children; this issue was central to its social investigation and policy recommendations. Dummer's convictions contrasted with this child-centered orientation and led her to define her projects and goals in some interesting ways. Specifically, her desire to ameliorate the harsh conditions surrounding motherhood led her to champion the rights of the most vulnerable and despised groups of mothers and the girls and women most likely to move into this category: unwed mothers, female delinquents, and prostitutes.

Dummer considered herself part of the maternal and infant welfare movement, and worked with and helped to fund the CB, but possessed a much more "rights-oriented"/feminist perspective than the progressive maternalists in the Bureau. That Dummer's political career encompassed an interest in female delinquency and sexuality, therefore, is not surprising. Unlike mainstream reproductive health activists, she acknowledged women's sexuality and its potential for both pleasure and danger. Therefore, Dummer's interest in maternal welfare, stemming from her feminism but not leading her directly toward the birth control movement as it did other feminists, illustrates another layer in the politics of maternal welfare.

The second half of this book shifts away from consideration of reformers associated with the CB to two women who were leaders in the birth control movement. In the same way that Dummer's and Putnam's careers help to contextualize the CB, Mary Ware Dennett and Blanche Ames add richness to our understanding of the politics of birth control in this crucial period that witnessed the nominal cultural and legal acceptance of artificial contraception.

The careers of Dennett and Ames illuminate more clearly the directions the mainstream movement took as well as the costs and payoffs of the compromises it made. Ames was a gentle and constructive critic of Margaret Sanger. The two women intermittently worked together and parted company when disagreements over strategy and ideology arose. Dennett's relations with Sanger were more contentious, as the latter two women strove to shape and lead the birth control movement in competing directions during the interwar years. Dennett's and Ames's distinct perspectives and tactics serve as counterpoints to Sanger's, offering new ways to assess both her great achievements and her misjudgments and mistakes.

Chapter 3 traces Mary Ware Dennett's political career in the birth control movement. Dennett's birth control work began when she helped establish the National Birth Control League (NBCL) in 1915. This event precipitated a contentious relationship between Dennett and Sanger, as the League was formed during the latter woman's flight from prosecution for violation of birth control statutes. For the next twenty years, Sanger and Dennett fought over the direction of the birth control movement in the United States. While Sanger was more interested in establishing clinics and passing legislation that would enable physicians to disseminate birth control, Dennett sought to ensure that birth control information and materials would be completely free from government interference or regulation. Dennett was the first of the two to move into the federal legislative arena by forming in 1919 the Voluntary Parenthood League, whose mission was reform of the federal obscenity statutes. Dennett continued to focus on ending government repression of scientific information throughout the 1920s, while Sanger, Ames, and others tried to steer clear of the civil liberties aspect of birth control to emphasize doctors' rights, women's health, and family stability. A birth control activist who promoted her cause neither as a feminist one nor a maternalist one, Dennett's career reveals the complexities of reproductive reform politics.

Blanche Ames was another birth control reformer whose career reflects the diversity of birth control politics and offers an instructive comparison to Sanger. Chapter 4 follows Ames's career and the fate of the birth control organizations she led in Massachusetts during the interwar years. Like Putnam, Ames was a wealthy, educated, and well-connected Boston reformer. Like Dennett, she prioritized birth control among the several causes that captured her attention in the interwar years. Her story is rife with frustrations and triumphs, and reveals the extent to which reproductive reform could be tackled from numerous vantage points over the course of an individual's career.

While Dennett led the first national birth control organization that attempted to tackle federal legislative reform, Ames counseled her state league to keep out of the federal arena. On the state level, the politics of birth control—negotiating the twists and turns of the judicial and legislative branches of local and national government—come to the foreground. Ames found that in her home state of Massachusetts a conservative climate necessitated deference to medical authority and a rejection of aggressive political tactics. Facing a conservative state legislature and a large local Catholic population, Massachusetts's birth control reformers chose to ally themselves with Sanger's American Birth Control League when convenient, but dropped their affiliation when it seemed politically appropriate. The story of the Massachusetts league reveals the multilayered politics of the birth control movement, its connection to maternal and infant welfare, and its ability to mutate into various forms and shapes according to the prevailing political environment.

1

"Maternity is not a contagious disease"

ELIZABETH LOWELL PUTNAM, PRENATAL CARE, AND CONSERVATIVE POLITICS

$\mathcal{I}n$ 1927, Elizabeth Putnam devised a devious plan to put the United States Children's Bureau (CB) out of operation permanently. She confided her secret to a high official in the United States Public Health Service, explaining, "I am gunning to be made chief of the Children's Bureau, in order that I may get that Bureau abolished without antagonism to the President from the women of the country."[1] Putnam audaciously followed through with her plan, asking President Calvin Coolidge to appoint her chief in 1928. Despite Putnam's prominence in the Republican Party and her notoriety as a pioneer in infant and maternal health, Coolidge felt compelled to refuse her request, pleading that such an appointment would be politically unfeasible. Putnam later divulged that President Coolidge admitted that, "he apparently had no way of getting rid of Grace Abbott."[2]

Putnam's hostility toward the CB was not unique in the 1920s, nor was her intention to have the Bureau abolished. The CB had been on shaky grounds since a conservative political climate and thrifty administration had been ushered in at the end of the First World War. However, Putnam's relationship to the CB was not nearly so simple as one of clear-cut enmity. On the contrary, Putnam was once a powerful ally to the Bureau, helping shape its early agenda and ensure its survival.

Elizabeth Lowell (1862–1935) was born in Brookline, Massachusetts, to August Lowell and Katherine Lawrence. Among the four siblings in her very prominent family were the poet Amy Lowell and Harvard President Abbott Lawrence Lowell. At the age of twenty-six, Elizabeth married William Lowell Putnam, a distinguished Boston lawyer and distant cousin. Putnam gave birth to five children, four of whom survived. Her two-year-old daughter Harriet died from drinking impure milk. This personal tragedy compelled Putnam to become active in the pure milk movement, from which she launched an impressive political career that consistently brought her into contact with the CB. Well connected, wealthy, and tenacious Putnam was a force to be reckoned with in Massachusetts and, increasingly, in the national political arena.

Significantly, Putnam's other pet cause in the first decades of the twentieth century was antisuffragism. She played an active role in the very powerful antisuffrage movement in Massachusetts. A political conservative, Putnam's desire to save the lives of babies and then their mothers through her work in the field of prenatal care did not reflect a commitment to equal rights for women. While this certainly separates her politically and ideologically from the other women reformers in this study and indeed the majority of reproductive reformers, Putnam does not represent an utterly unique case. Indeed, her eclectic political commitments reflected the power of reproductive issues to attract those from the right as well as those from the left.[3]

Despite her adamant opposition to women's suffrage, Putnam was a dedicated political activist from 1908, when she first joined and chaired the executive committee of the Massachusetts Milk Consumers' Association, until her death in 1935. Putnam rose to prominence in reform circles just prior to World War I. In 1909—the same year as the White House Conference on the Care of Dependent Children—she initiated a five-year study of the effects of prenatal care on infant mortality. Her work brought her national recognition as a lay expert in this field. Among the many reproductive health organizations she led or participated in were the American Association for the Study and Prevention of Infant Mortality, the Women's Municipal League of Boston, the American Child Hygiene Association, the Household Nursing Association, and the National Child Welfare Association.

Like many elite women in the early twentieth century—both liberals and conservatives—Putnam was enabled by the politics of maternalism to launch and legitimate a political career. According to Seth Koven and Sonya Michel, maternalism refers to "ideologies and discourses that exalted women's capacity to mother and applied to society as a whole the values they attached to that role: care, nurturance, and morality."[4] Significantly, Putnam's maternalism offered a way into both the antisuffrage and the infant welfare movements. As the chair of the education and organizing committee of the Women's Anti-Suffrage Association of Massachusetts, for example, Putnam wrote: "Woman is the bearer and rearer of children. Mercifully no suffrage agitation can deprive her of this privilege. Her first duty must

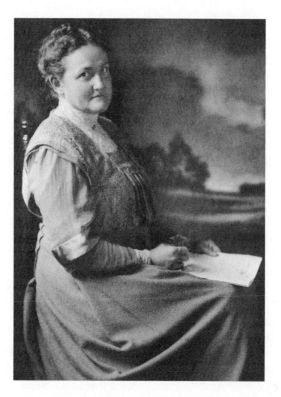

FIG. 1 ELIZABETH LOWELL PUTNAM.
Photo courtesy of the Schlesinger Library, Radcliffe
Institute, Harvard University.

always be at home and her best effort must be given to her home and what makes for the betterment of homes the world over. . . . A woman wields immense power just because she has no political affiliations"[5]

To accomplish their goals, the maternalists with whom historians are most familiar—progressive maternalists—engaged in a conscious battle to transform the liberal state into an activist one. Or, put another way, "they transformed motherhood from women's primary *private* responsibility into *public* policy."[6] While Putnam certainly shared the desire to come to the aid of mothers and infants, she increasingly opposed the methods of mainstream reformers.

Putnam's career and ideology, representative of a much larger conservative movement, help us understand how opposition to welfare state development was compatible with reproductive reform. An examination of the choices, alliances, and enemies Putnam made during her thirty years of activism provides a clear illustration of the extent to which a desire to help women and children during their most vulnerable life stages (pregnancy and infancy) could conflict with government initiatives to aid maternal health. While Putnam dedicated herself to saving the lives of infants and mothers, she increasingly saw the CB as a competitor for power and authority and as fundamentally misguided. Her career forces historians to rethink the contributions of conservative, politically active, and powerful women in the development of public policy. Her activities and ideology pose the question of how a conservative political agenda could be meshed with an innovative reform spirit and a sincere concern for women and children.[7]

In addition to the fact that Putnam's career illuminates the variable ways that maternalism intersected with what Koven has called "a wide array of concrete social and political practices," it serves as a foil to the history of the CB. By contrast, Putnam helps to expose both the flaws in the CB's orientation, and its great strengths and achievements. For example, Linda Gordon and others have argued that the weakness of social welfare programs in this country has stemmed partially from a gendered conception of social provision versus social assistance. Gordon has been critical of the way in which women's social work heritage has led to an emphasis on treatment for poor people, rather than prevention of poverty.[8] Putnam's reform career shows that, in the case of reproductive reform politics, concern for the poor, whether communicated through advocacy of treatment or prevention, cannot be taken for granted. The lengths that the CB went to to ameliorate the suffering of disadvantaged groups need to be evaluated not only in the light of more advanced and progressive activities (as we will do in the next chapter when considering Ethel Dummer), but in relation to more conservative actions as well. Putnam, once an ally and increasingly an outspoken critic of the CB, helps to underscore the variety of paths available to white middle-class women who shared a desire to improve the welfare of mothers and their babies.

I have identified three distinct phases of Putnam's dynamic reform career dating from 1908 to her death in 1935. In the first phase, dating roughly from 1908 to 1920, Putnam's maternalism provided the most important organizing principle in her politics. Although she was a political conservative who vigorously opposed women's suffrage, her maternalism allowed her to cross many boundaries to become a prominent figure in the predominantly progressive circles of the infant welfare movement. She enjoyed status and fame among the ranks of reformers, the loss of which would plague her throughout the last decade of her life.

The second phase of Putnam's career began with the passage of the Sheppard-Towner Act, and the appointment of Grace Abbott as chief of the CB in 1921, and lasted three or four years. During these years, Putnam's conservative political orientation vied for supremacy over her maternalism as she made a break from various progressive welfare organizations and became an outspoken critic of Sheppard-Towner. In this second, transitional period, Putnam's opposition to Sheppard-Towner grew less out of a critique of the welfare state than out of particular problems she had with the administration and administrators of the new federal program. She kept her antagonisms directed at specific political issues and people, and maintained that there were more efficient ways to help women and children than through the plan devised by the CB.

Putnam's growing interest in attaining status and power within the Republican Party also marked this second phase. Once the Nineteenth Amendment passed, Putnam was not shy about exercising her new rights, and even sought official positions within the party apparatus. By 1920, many reformers had bolted from the Republican Party to support first the Progressive Party and, ultimately, the Democrats. Putnam, however, remained loyal to the Republican Party as it developed a more conservative constituency and agenda in the 1920s.

The third and final phase of Putnam's political career began in the mid- to late 1920s when her conservatism virtually eclipsed her maternalism. She ceased being a careful and considerate critic of particular methods and agencies in the national infant welfare movement. Instead, she initiated a wholesale attack on federal "paternalism" and the very existence of the CB. In this final period, Putnam lost all her previous connections to maternal and infant health care reformers and actually formed her own right-wing women's organization "to abolish the Children's Bureau . . . and to stifle other welfare legislation affecting mothers and children."[9] She also became a member of the archconservative group the Sentinels of the Republic, which supported and encouraged her disassociation from her previous reform affiliations. Thus, Putnam's reform career had come full circle. While maternalism had initially proved a bridge across different political orientations, by the end of the 1920s debates about the role of the federal government had come to the foreground and cost Putnam her prominent place in the maternal and infant welfare movement. This chapter will trace the development of Putnam's reform career and show her shifting priorities and networks throughout the three phases I have identified, highlighting the ideological distance that grew between Putnam and the CB.

THE MAKING OF A CONSERVATIVE MATERNALIST: PUTNAM'S FIRST STAGE OF ACTIVISM

Putnam was an important pioneer and participant in what historian Richard A. Meckel has categorized as the second and third stages of the infant welfare movement in the United States. Meckel has argued that interest in lowering the infant mortality rate in the United States passed through three distinct phases. The first, lasting from approximately 1850 to 1880, marked the "discovery" of the high infant mortality rate by reformers. The second phase lasted from the 1880s through the 1910s and focused on the importance of infant nutrition, specifically, on debating the pros and cons of breast versus "artificial" feeding. The third phase began in the first decade of the twentieth century and defined infant welfare primarily in terms of motherhood, dually focusing on women's health during pregnancy, and educating women to mother properly.

The earliest infant welfare reformers tended to look toward the environment as the perpetuator of disease. Sanitary reformers dominated the ranks in this first stage of the infant welfare movement. They recognized that child rearing customs and medical treatment needed to be examined, but believed that only through changing the environmental conditions in which infants lived would a drastic improvement be made in mortality rates. Thus, early infant welfare work concentrated on municipal and sanitary reforms such as housing reform to increase sunlight and air circulation and to lessen numbers of people living under one roof; efforts to expedite the effective removal of garbage; and attempts to improve the availability and cleanliness of water and fuel. But, as immigrants continued to crowd into large urban centers, there seemed little hope for turning back the clock toward a more traditional, healthy environment for infants and their families.

By the 1880s reformers narrowed their focus to infant nutrition, specifically, artificial feeding. Meckel has argued that this narrower focus was accepted by the scientific, medical, and lay community because it provided a reasonable scientific explanation of infant mortality, and "also promised a solution to the dilemma that public health reformers had found themselves facing in their attempts to reduce mortality among urban infants."[10] For the first time scientists were able to make accurate bacteria counts in cows' milk. They found that commercial milk was a breeding ground for the bacteria and germs that led to the primary cause of infant death: the infant diarrhea epidemic common to children in urban areas in the summer months. Thus, the most logical and efficient way to proceed would be to clean up the milk supply.

Infant welfare reform, and milk reform in particular, remained at the local level throughout the nineteenth and into the first decades of the twentieth centuries. Municipalities took the lead in passing milk laws. Between 1880 and 1895, twenty-three U.S. cities passed or reinforced legislation related to safeguarding their milk supply.[11] However, most municipalities received their milk from the countryside, which was outside their jurisdiction and the place where most of the adulteration was thought to occur. After this discovery it became necessary to involve the state apparatus in the regulatory process. Milk dealers protested the regulatory function of local governments. Ironically, these challenges often led to an increase in the authority of local governments in the arena of public health. Meckel asserts, "The court challenges that dealers and retailers mounted against health departments produced a series of federal and state court decisions that eventually established the power of city health officials to regulate the sale of milk within their municipal borders, even if it was produced outside."[12] Thus, in the second phase of the infant welfare movement, the milk question was closely associated with debates over the role of the government in regulating trade and protecting public health.

Putnam's entrance into the world of reform coincided with Meckel's second phase of the infant welfare movement. Her activity in the pure milk movement (and her consequent commitment to infant welfare reform in all its forms) was almost certainly inspired by the death of her infant daughter, Harriet, as a result of drinking unclean milk. Putnam's initial political activity developed from her membership in a civic group, the Women's Municipal League of Boston, within which she formed a separate Committee on Milk in 1908. Two years later she joined the Massachusetts Milk Consumers' Association (MMCA). The MMCA's aim was to "unite consumers in obtaining efficient inspection and a pure milk supply" in order to reduce infant mortality and prevent epidemics among the larger population.[13] This organization's commitment to consumers signaled a path that would be well-worn by Putnam.

Both the MMCA and the Committee on Milk of the Women's Municipal League dedicated themselves to passing legislation to insure efficient and adequate inspection of the state milk supply. In the battle for improved milk inspection, Putnam found herself on the bad side of businessmen, and even local boards of health that feared intrusion into their domain. In a letter to the editor of the *Worcester Telegram* on October 6, 1911, regarding the pure milk bill that was currently before the state legislature, Putnam wrote, "There is no ground whatever for saying that the bill is . . . an effort to destroy local government. . . . It simply provides for a central, coordinating authority to make sure that the field is completely covered and to save uneconomical and annoying duplication of inspection. In other words, it puts a general at the head of the army for the prevention of disease, the individual units of the army being the local boards of health which still continue to do their work under the Ellis Bill."[14] In her advocacy of centralization, a scientific approach to social problems, and her critique of entrepreneurial freedom when it came into conflict with adequate safeguards for public health, Putnam articulates several key tenets of progressivism. Continuing her editorial, Putnam claimed, "The rights of the innocent consumer to protection from disease and death, so far outweigh any possible rights to manufacture such disease and death, however innocently, that the public need only to understand the facts in order to insist on this protection."[15]

Particular features of Massachusetts's politics and public health history can help explain Putnam's ostensibly progressive position on the milk question. Politically, Massachusetts boasted a long history of regulation of commerce in the interest of the public good. According to Massachusetts historian Barbara Gutman Rosenkrantz, "Civic responsibility to protect 'the public interest' from ignorance, irresponsibility, or selfishness—whatever its source—had long been assumed by successive generations of enlightened Republicans whose candidates for public office were drawn from the old stock of native Americans."[16] This group of old stock Americans from whom Putnam's prominent family drew its power and exerted its influence certainly shaped Putnam's growing political interests. Specifically in the arena of public health, the Massachusetts Board of Health was run by a group of scientists who argued that they "should have principal responsibility for direct hygienic intervention to promote public health."[17] By 1890, the state's responsibility and obligation to prevent the contamination of the public water supply was firmly established in Massachusetts. Once a scientific consensus developed around methods for controlling water-borne diseases, the Massachusetts Board of Health "took the lead in pointing to the protection of milk as the next critical area for the promotion of public health."[18] Board scientists began to count the bacteria in the Boston milk supply as early as 1890. Endorsing the motto, "Be Clean," the Board called for restrictive laws that "required individual vigilance at every point from the farmer to the consumer."[19]

Like the settlement house workers and club women she then associated with, Putnam followed a trajectory from the municipal to the state and, eventually, to the federal reform arena. Her activity in the pure milk movement in Massachusetts led her to advocate not only state regulation of the milk supply, but also cooperation between federal and state inspectors. Although she received little encouragement, Putnam even wrote requesting an audience with President William Howard Taft in 1909 so that she might urge him to facilitate such an association. She wrote, "Both the United States Pure Food Commission and our own Health Authorities tell me that by cooperating they could do much more than is at present possible to purify Boston's milk supply. Very unfortunately, however, there has been . . . little of such cooperation."[20] Putnam never received an audience with Taft. He directed her comments and suggestions to the Pure Food Commission and the Public Health Service.

Putnam's activities and strategies in the MMCA complemented those of women progressives who also sought to improve social conditions through both government regulation and consumer education and activism. Florence Kelley's work with the National Consumers' League (NCL) (founded in 1899 by Josephine Shaw Lowell) provides a good example. In later years Kelley would become the victim of Putnam's political red baiting and the latter would vehemently deny any suggestion of commonalties in methods or goals. Under the leadership of Florence Kelley from its founding until her death in 1932, the NCL lobbied for social welfare and labor legislation at the state and federal levels. Both the NCL and the smaller MMCA aimed to regulate aspects of the production of goods and services through the power of the organized and educated consumer. However, Kelley's concern lay with disadvantaged groups. Through the NCL she sought to harness the power of consumers to protect exploited factory and sweated workers. In the field of infant welfare, Kelley and her Hull House compatriots focused on making clean milk available to poor families in urban areas through milk stations. Putnam, less interested in milk stations, fought to have a clean milk supply available to consumers. Her concern was the consumer, not the power consumers held over the conditions of production. The key distinction between these strategies lay in their aims: to improve either access to or provision of goods and services. While Putnam's work emphasized the former, liberals and socialists sought to tackle the latter. Putnam sought to make clean milk available for purchase, while advocates of milk stations went a step further to ensure that milk would reach those in need.[21] This early difference in perspective foreshadowed problems that would later develop between Putnam and those Progressives she cooperated with in the prewar period. For the time being, though, Putnam and other infant welfare reformers used compatible, if not identical, tactics to lower infant mortality rates through regulation of the milk supply.

Another commonality between Putnam and her more progressive colleagues lay in the rhetorical strategies they employed. According to Kathryn Kish Sklar, "as head of the NCL, Kelley exemplified the moral conclusions to be drawn from infant mortality statistics collected by the U.S. Children's Bureau, when in 1920 she repeatedly demanded on behalf of the Sheppard-Towner Act, 'why does Congress wish Babies to die?'"[22] Putnam similarly never let the public forget the helpless babies who were the victims of the unclean milk supply. In a Women's Municipal League Bulletin from 1912, Putnam's words ironically presage Kelley's statement in support of Sheppard-Towner: "Already since the veto last year it is safe to say that at least 3000 lives have been lost which might have been saved, and this number is increasing yearly. Is it not time we rouse ourselves? It is public opinion, public help that is needed. The politicians would not play politics with the lives of little children if they were made to feel that people cared about this thing."[23] This type of rhetoric was useful for Putnam's pure milk campaign because it roused public opinion and, more specifically, appealed to the women reformers in the General Federation of Women's Clubs (GFWC), which by the end of the decade had close to one million members.

From 1909, when Putnam first published an article in the *Federation Bulletin* (the official organ of the GFWC) on the milk question, until the early teens, Putnam made a special effort to receive endorsements from this umbrella organization. In 1912 she wrote to the president of the Massachusetts branch of the federated clubs and asked if there was anything she could do "to rouse interest in the Federated Women's Clubs." She offered to "come before your gathering ready to answer any questions which any of your members might ask."[24] Two years later, when Putnam's energy was focused almost entirely on improving prenatal care, she would again count on the GFWC for support. In a discussion of how to get patients to enter prenatal care programs presented to the American Association for the Study and Prevention of Infant Mortality in November 1914, Putnam acknowledged the power of organized womanhood and women's special connection to this issue: "It seems to me that one of the most fruitful ways and one in which I am personally much interested is through the Federated Women's Clubs. There are enormous numbers of women belonging to these clubs now and it certainly is a woman's job to take care of herself and her children; consequently these clubs are admirably adapted to take up this work. I believe if the women's clubs throughout the country could be roused to the need of proper prenatal and obstetrical care, the battle would be won, and I think it should not be difficult thing to do."[25] The same year that Putnam sought alliance with women's clubs, the GFWC decided to endorse women's suffrage. One year later, in 1915, the Massachusetts suffrage referendum would suffer a great defeat due to the power of organized antisuffragism in the state.

Despite conflict among female reformers over women's suffrage, however, Putnam was able to make connection with these women through the shared politics of maternalism. In addition to soliciting the cooperation of the GFWC, Putnam's milk politics were endorsed by such diverse groups as the Massachusetts State Branch of the American Federation of Labor and the Massachusetts Medical Society.

In 1909, Putnam branched out from her primary focus on milk to begin an innovative prenatal care experiment. Putnam established a small-scale prenatal care clinic for middle-class women in Boston to discern the efficacy of this type of care. Putnam's shift in emphasis was part of a larger movement among infant welfare reformers in the first decades of the twentieth century. This shift toward focusing on mothers to save babies opened up a debate not only about child rearing but forced attention on pregnancy itself, ultimately leading reformers to concentrate on prenatal care. Efforts to improve prenatal care took various routes; the three principle methods were education, financial assistance, and improvements in medical care. Education proved the most popular strategy for U.S. reformers, as it could sidestep delicate questions of poverty and the socioeconomic aspects of infant mortality. Many reformers who wished to improve access to health care without redistributing resources in any permanent sense saw maternal education as a great leveler.

Putnam's experiment of providing prenatal care to middle-class women went a step beyond the general efforts to educate women, although its narrow class orientation necessarily weakened its ultimate legacy. Putnam's intent was to prove that proper prenatal care given by visiting nurses and regular obstetrical examinations could drastically reduce instances of both infant and maternal mortality. At the end of her five-year experiment, 1,522 babies were successfully delivered; no women died during pregnancy and less than 1 percent died at confinement; there were .2 percent miscarriages; and 2.8 percent of the babies died at under one month of age. These averages were considerably lower then national averages.[26] By 1915 the Women's Municipal League had three clinics: the original one started at the Peter Brent Brigham Hospital, a clinic at the Maverick Dispensary in East Boston, and one at the Cambridge Neighborhood House.

The efforts of the Women's Municipal League were not philanthropic, but intentionally aimed at the middle class. Putnam insured that the clinics would address the needs of middle-class women by charging between five and ten dollars per patient during the first year of the experiment. Afterwards, a sliding scale was developed before another reorganization of the clinic system in cooperation with local hospitals in 1917. Putnam aimed to make the clinics self-supporting so as to ensure their survival. In addition to this pragmatic reason, Putnam's political beliefs led her away from charitable work. She argued, "we believe that self-supporting work is of far more value than that supported by charity—for not only is there no limit to growth, but it is much more appreciated by those who benefit from it."[27]

Putnam and her committee argued that the middle class was "the class in the community always least well cared for."[28] Putnam explained, "The rich can afford the best care and to the poor—a very large number of the poor—it is given free in the clinics of the best hospitals; but the women whose margin of income over output is small are terribly apt to get into the hands of those whose knowledge of the proper care to be given in pregnancy and at confinement leaves much to be desired."[29] Putnam's characterization of the local obstetrical scene surely glossed over some significant class dynamics in health care provision. Specifically, her confidence that the poor were receiving care in the best hospital clinics needs to be qualified. Although early-twentieth-century obstetricians may have been pleased "to have charity patients whose reproductive processes they might observe with a steady, clinical eye," these same doctors tended to view this population "as defective both in health and moral ability, and thus in greater need of assistance from medical arts than were healthy and respectable women."[30] Once again, as in the case of milk stations, Putnam displays a cavalier attitude regarding the circumstances of the poor, and in particular poor pregnant women and mothers.

Ironically, the narrow class focus of Putnam's activities exempted her from the problems and complications inherent in much cross-class social welfare activity. In attempting to provide an innovative service for women more like herself in terms of economic background, Putnam avoided the many pitfalls of cross-class social welfare work. Because she believed through her clinic she was helping a more educated class of women, her work did not carry undertones of paternalism, nor did she aim at control of another class or ethnic group. Her activities on behalf of middle-class women remind us that sensitivity toward and concern for the poor were not inextricably linked with reproductive health reform. While much work on social welfare reformers has emphasized their class, race, and ethnic biases or prejudices, their dedication to the disadvantaged classes should not be taken for granted.[31]

Before United States involvement in World War I, the Women's Municipal League clinics were successful in their efforts to help a limited population, but they remained small. Once war was declared, the medical director of the original Peter Brent Brigham clinic joined the Medical

Reserve corps and the clinic was closed temporarily. By August 1917, the Women's Municipal League, in affiliation with the outpatient department of the Peter Brent Brigham Hospital and the staff of the Boston Lying-In Hospital, reopened its largest and most successful clinic. Patients were responsible for the cost of both the doctor and nurse as well as any clinic charges as, once again, a primary goal of the project was to make the clinic entirely self-supporting. Putnam was pleased with the new arrangement of the clinic, as it went even further to ensure a middle-class clientele. She argued, "The most immediately interesting development is that we have already more patients coming to the clinic than we had before when they were not paying nearly the expense of their care. The results are exceedingly gratifying, for they go to show that the clinic is meeting a real need, and that we are . . . really at last getting hold of the great class of people of very moderate means."[32]

Putnam's intent was to reach a section of the population that she believed was overlooked by physicians. Significantly, her prenatal care experiment was conducted prior to the CB studies that showed that mortality decreased as family income rose. Thus, although logic and sensitivity would seem to have directed attention to those in poverty, Putnam's belief that middle-class women were most in need of services was not contradicted by statistical evidence at this point.

The Women's Municipal League clinics gained patients and notoriety over the next few years. Putnam used the opportunity of this success to promote her cause as well as herself. The cooperation of Brigham and Boston Lying-In Hospitals as well as dispensaries and settlement houses clearly attests to the immediate influence of Putnam's vision on the local infant and maternal welfare movement. The fact that Putnam's audience was made up largely of liberal social workers calls attention to the critical role she played in the development of prenatal care in Boston and its discovery and acceptance on a national scale. Therefore, it is not surprising that she chose Paul Kellogg's *Survey* as a forum to publish an article on her prenatal care experiment.

In her 1914 article entitled "Prenatal Care of the Next Generation," Putnam began to establish herself publicly as a pioneer and expert in the field of prenatal care. She argued that, due to the Women's Municipal League experiment, the Boston Lying-In Hospital had established its own clinic with a visiting nurse to carry out prenatal work. In addition, Putnam contended that there was a direct causal relationship between the Women's Municipal League experiment and the Boston Board of Health's decision in 1911 to send two nurses throughout the city to care for mothers and babies. By 1913, the Board of Health was employing ten

visiting nurses. Putnam was particularly pleased that "A permanent committee consisting of obstetricians, social workers, and trained nurses has
also been formed in Boston to standardize and coordinate all prenatal work
being done in the city, to the end that it shall be as customary for all women
as care is now at the moment of birth."[33] This triumvirate of doctors, social
workers, and nurses exemplified the kind of holistic approach to maternal
and infant welfare that we most closely associate with the CB. Robyn
Muncy characterizes this approach most succinctly when she writes,
"Women in the child welfare corps . . . defined maternal and infant mortality as a multi-faceted social problem requiring the attention of specialists in
medicine, social economics, sanitation, nutrition, education, industrial
safety, city planning, home economics, and law. . . . An agency filled with
social workers, doctors, nurses, teachers, home economists, and nutrition-
ists would better address maternal and infant mortality than a bureau of
doctors, who would take too narrow a view of the issue to study its fullest
causes."[34] By the end of the decade, this holistic approach would be pitted
against a purely medical orientation in the struggle over Sheppard-Towner,
and Putnam would side decisively with doctors. For now, though, she supported an approach to prenatal care that included the likes of social workers
as well as physicians. Furthermore, in her advocacy of a central coordinating
agency and her efforts to bring science and efficiency to prenatal care
throughout the city, Putnam's orientation still seems close to that of her progressive colleagues. However, the fault line that began to grow stemmed
from Putnam's lack of concern for charitable work. As in her disdain for
milk stations, Putnam wanted improved prenatal care to be available, but
was less interested in which populations of women would have access to it.

Putnam possessed a vision of maternity and infant care that included
respect for the mother's life and well-being and respect for the responsibilities of motherhood. Like many reformers in this period, her commitment to infant welfare had led her to maternity and the discovery that
maternal mortality represented an equally appalling problem. Putnam's
hopes for a future filled with more humane treatment of mothers can be
found in one of her addresses regarding the prenatal care experiment:

> In trying to reach women with such a clinic as this, one suffers from the fact
> that childbearing is such an ancient function. Women have suffered and
> died in childbirth since the beginning, and they expect to go on giving their
> lives for the life of the race to the end of time . . . ignorant that much of the
> suffering and the greater number of deaths from this natural function are
> entirely unnecessary. The knowledge of better conditions is like a snow
> ball—the greater it becomes, the faster it rolls up, but the effort to start the

ball rolling is heart-breaking in its slowness when one realizes the intense need for it.[35]

Once again, her progressive spirit reveals itself as she pits herself against forces that would bow to the inevitability of maternal death. Putnam sought to use knowledge, particularly scientific knowledge, to improve women's chances of survival and railed against the martyrdom associated with motherhood.

Putnam's enthusiasm and compassion as a reformer was as highly regarded as her practical and scientific expertise in the prewar years. By 1918 she had written, co-authored, or edited close to a dozen articles on the subject of maternal and infant welfare. Through her leadership in the Women's Municipal League's Committee on Infant Social Services (which later became the Committee on Prenatal and Obstetrical Care) Putnam forged ties with infant welfare activists across the political spectrum. While later in her life she would rail against the settlement house mentality and, specifically, the radicalism of the Hull House group, in 1912 she happily reported to the Women's Municipal League that "we have got into most pleasant relations with all prenatal workers in Boston through a meeting held at South End House in January."[36] In this early phase of her career Putnam enjoyed cordial relations with the social workers at both South End House and the Cambridge Neighborhood House, the latter being one of the sites of a Women's Municipal League prenatal care clinic.

In addition to creating a congenial network among her Bostonian colleagues, Putnam's prewar activities and expertise attracted national attention. In May 1913, Putnam participated in a Baby Saving Show in Philadelphia, which she helped organize. Organizations that requested information on prenatal care from Putnam from 1909 through 1913 (before the results of her five year experiment were even available) included the Child Welfare Committee, New York City; the Bureau of Municipal Research, Philadelphia; the Maryland Association for the Study and Prevention of Infant Mortality; the Babies Milk Fund Association of Louisville, Kentucky; the Infant Welfare Society of Chicago; the Toronto Department of Health; the Child Hygiene Association of Philadelphia; and the United Jewish Educational and Charitable Association of St. Louis, Missouri.

In 1918 Putnam's national reputation was solidified when she became president of the American Association for the Study and Prevention of Infant Mortality (AASPIM). This groundbreaking organization was founded in 1909 by reformers devoted to treating infant mortality as a multifaceted social problem. With its formation, "what had been an inchoate movement, consisting of the uncoordinated and little publicized efforts of various individuals, urban health departments, and voluntary agencies, gained a national forum and a promotional organization."[37]

During this stage of her career, Putnam displayed no compunctions about using municipal and state governments to serve her cause. Eager to clean up the milk supply and promote prenatal care, she worked for government regulation and bureaucratic expansion. She confirmed her connections to the infant and maternal welfare movement through her efforts to pass a Massachusetts Maternity Bill in 1920. The bill, "An Act to Provide Adequate Care for Mothers and Children During the Maternity Period," placed the department of public health in charge of administering maternal and infant health care. The bill authorized the Department of Public Health, "To furnish, in addition to advice and instruction, nursing and expert prenatal care to pregnant women at home, at some hospital or local clinic at the option of the expectant mother, also nursing or hospital care at the time of confinement if in the judgment of said department the safety of mother of child requires such care."[38] The bill was introduced by laywomen reformers, but had the approval of the State Department of Public Health, the department that would administer the measure. The legislative committee of the Massachusetts Medical Society, the Massachusetts Homeopathic Medical Society, and the State Federation of Women's Clubs also approved the bill. Despite the inclusion of the pro-suffrage women's clubs among its supporters, Putnam actively involved herself with its passage, lobbying before the Committee on Rules of the Massachusetts House of Representatives. She received a letter from a member of the Rules Committee complimenting her on the statement that she made on maternity care at the hearings the month before. He wrote that he had "never heard a more convincing speech."[39]

Putnam not only spoke before the Rules Committee on the importance of prenatal care, but she also wrote letters to various politicians in support of the bill. Writing to Lieutenant Governor Frank G. Allen in May 1920, Putnam spoke of her immense interest in the passage of the maternity aid bill, quoted the latest maternal mortality statistics, and, finally, enclosed literature on her own prenatal care experiment from 1909 through 1914. She established herself as both a concerned citizen and an expert in the field. Putnam was convinced that the state of Massachusetts needed to involve itself with the health of its mothers and children. She argued that "this bill should do much toward starting in this community a different standard for the care of women in childbirth with an attendant great reduction of the death rate. Massachusetts has always been in the lead—let us keep her there."[40]

Perhaps the most convincing evidence of Putnam's close association with her more progressive colleagues throughout the first two decades of the twentieth century was her cordial, cooperative, and supportive relationship with Julia Lathrop and the staff of the CB. At the very start of her career as chief of the newly created federal CB, Julia Lathrop wrote to Putnam asking for her cooperation in developing the agenda of the Bureau. Putnam's input was eagerly sought in an effort to make the CB's first publication *Prenatal Care* both up-to-date and successful. Mary Mills West sent Putnam a draft of her bulletin on prenatal care, along with a self-addressed, stamped envelope for her comments. West wrote, "Would it be asking too much of you to beg you to look it over and let me know what you think of it, and of its usefulness? If there is someone else whom you would like to ask to read it will you not do so? . . . I beg you to believe that we shall regard your attention as a great service to the Bureau."[41] In a letter to West in March 1913, just after receiving a copy of *Prenatal Care,* Putnam wrote, "It seems to me a remarkably clear and well balanced statement of all the circumstances, and I like to think what an era it will make—it makes me so proud of your Bureau!"[42] In an effort to include as many women as possible in this revolutionary new era of prenatal care, Putnam suggested to West that she should include "Something really short suited to the comparatively uneducated and the poor if this seems feasible."[43] However, Putnam's generous spirit only extended as far as advocating free advice, and not to more expensive medical treatment.

In addition to seeking her input on their publications, both Lathrop and West asked Putnam for advice and guidance in their many varied pursuits. They sought to learn as much as possible from her five-year experiment. In the first year of her administration Lathrop wrote, "The work which you have undertaken in prenatal care we recognize as very important, and we desire to have someone from the Bureau visit Boston and see it at first-hand."[44] Indeed, Lathrop eventually asked Putnam to send the CB "all possible information about your work" in the Women's Municipal League.[45] Before Putnam's conservative politics would create an insurmountable barrier between them, Lathrop even expected her help in drafting the CB's innovative questionnaire used in its local studies of infant mortality. "This schedule, or questionnaire, is sent you, knowing your deep personal interest in the general problem, in the hope that you will examine it with what care your time will permit, with a view to your suggesting to the Bureau such modifications as you would recommend either in scope, or in the scheme itself."[46]

Putnam's reaction to this type of inquiry was extremely positive. She wrote to Lathrop one week later, using this opportunity to praise the

Bureau and to add her own commentary on the milk question:

> I am so glad you are finding out why babies lives as well as why they die. We focus our attention too much on sick babies. If the time and money we spend on sickness were devoted to keeping people well, much more would be accomplished, and incidentally if that spent on milk stations were given to improving the quality of the general milk supply, so that all the people could buy decently clean milk . . . the community would be immensely more benefited. Milk stations as such, are a confession of failure, but the visiting nurses they employ are the salvation of the poor.[47]

Although Putnam's emphasis on prevention was in keeping with the Bureau's own philosophy, her skepticism about milk stations repudiated a long-standing philanthropic tradition.[48] In assuming that, once pure milk was made available, it could readily be obtained by all consumers, Putnam exposed a notable insensitivity to the poor that would later contribute to her alienation from the Bureau and from mainstream child and maternal welfare reformers. For the time being, however, Putnam enthusiastically praised the Bureau's approach to the problem of infant mortality and welfare.

The staff of the CB had found a powerful ally in Elizabeth Putnam. She was a prominent, well-connected, and active citizen even before the right to vote was thrust upon her in 1920. While the staff of the CB did not look to her for philanthropic contributions, they knew they could benefit from her expertise and political connections.

Putnam's support of the CB did not end with her consultations. She also helped the Bureau in its political struggle to stay alive in the early years. In April 1914, Putnam wrote to senators and representatives on the Committee on Ways and Means on behalf of the CB at the request of the National Child Labor Committee's Owen Lovejoy: "Will you kindly do all that you can to help pass the appropriation of $165,000 asked for by the CB? They have done excellent work and ought to be encouraged instead of having their appropriations cut down. This work happens to be one in which I am personally very much interested, so that I speak whereof I know as to their work."[49] In her presidential address at the ninth annual meeting of the AASPIM in 1918 (which in the same year changed its name to the American Child Hygiene Association) in Chicago, Putnam continued to publicly support and praise the activities of the CB. "The weighing plan of the CB is doing pioneering educational work in awakening the mothers of the present generation to the needs of the generation just starting on the road."[50]

Even after being chief of the CB for seven years, Lathrop still forwarded requests for information to Putnam. In 1919, for example, Putnam received a letter forwarded from the CB on behalf of the Italian Branch of the International Council of Women. This organization requested information on mothers' pensions, prenatal care, milk inspection, and free medical care for young children and pregnant women. Putnam provided the Italian women's group with literature chronicling the work of the Women's Municipal League and the Massachusetts Milk Consumers Association. Although the CB had by this time published its own very successful bulletins on *Prenatal Care* and *Infant Care*, Lathrop continued to utilize Putnam's personal expertise.[51]

The relationship between Putnam and the CB was not entirely one-sided. Putnam utilized her relations with the Bureau to promote her own work. For example, in December 1917, as president of the AASPIM, Putnam sought funds from the Rockefeller Foundation to continue the Association's prenatal work. The Foundation asked Putnam to describe the Associations's relations with the CB and implied that a positive letter of evaluation from Julia Lathrop would reflect the worthiness of the AASPIM's request. Putnam asked Lathrop for her endorsement, and wrote to Dr. George Vincent of the Rockefeller Foundation, "I should like to say that my own relations could hardly be pleasanter or more satisfactory then they are with Miss Lathrop and her staff."[52] In turn, Lathrop provided Putnam with a letter of recommendation that praised the "invaluable educational services" provided by the AASPIM, especially in regard to Children's Year, and pointed to the need for "public and private effort together to do all the work conserving . . . infancy and childhood."[53] Indeed, Putnam's relationship with the CB seemed mutually advantageous in this period. The Bureau received information and endorsements from a prominent citizen and lay expert, and Putnam expanded the scope of her authority within the reform community.

☙❦❧

Putnam's prominence in the field of maternal and infant welfare gave her numerous opportunities to associate with more liberal reproductive reformers. As we have already seen, before 1921, her antisuffrage position did not hamper her from cooperating with the federated women's clubs or the first chief of the U.S. Children's Bureau; nor did she shy away from involvement with local settlement houses. Putnam received requests for speeches, articles, and information regularly throughout the first phase of her career. Requests for her services and support came even from the still small and decidedly progressive birth control movement. At this issue Putnam drew the line. Despite her commitment to improving the next generation, Putnam professed revulsion towards artificial birth control. Putnam's lack of support for birth control is unremarkable, reflecting the mainstream consensus among reproductive health reformers in the interwar years. But the lengths to which birth control reformers went to gain her support are remarkable in the context of her conservative reputation.

According to one historian, "The antisuffrage role in the birth control controversy was to call attention to what they regarded as the sinister relationship between women's suffrage and birth control."[54] Putnam used this particular tactic in a letter to the editor of the *New York Post* in 1916 when she wrote: "The public press is teeming with birth control and woman suffrage. If women and men both were taught to practice self-control, the hysteria about birth control, both for and against, would die of inanition, and if women would study the world in which they live from the point of view of the world, rather than of self, many of the fancied suffragists would drop away. The time in which we are living is too big with the future to be spent in pettiness."[55] Most suffragists would balk at the association of their cause with birth control, as many agreed that it represented either a selfish desire on the part of women or an effort to elude responsibility on the part of men.[56] However, savvy political activists like Putnam sought to taint women's suffrage with the stigma of birth control.

In 1918, Putnam publicly addressed the issue of birth control in her presidential address to the AASPIM. She caricatured the movement as "saying to people, 'Do what you like and as much of it as you like and I'll show you how to get away with it.'"[57] Despite these strong words, Putnam went on to say, "I do not want to be understood to mean that there are no conditions under which the control of conception in ways other than by total abstention is justifiable, but that the irresponsible manner of their preachment by the advocates of 'birth control' is dangerous to the community."[58] In bringing up the issue of birth control and then admitting that she had reservations about total prohibition of the practice, Putnam placed herself in a controversial position within her reform community. Indeed, her decision to mention the topic in her presidential address with less than total disapproval marks her sincerity in confronting, if not accepting the broad scope of ideas that made up reproductive reform.

One of the principal reasons for Putnam's acknowledgment of the birth control issue was her receipt on a fairly regular basis of correspondence from various birth control reformers and organizations. In September

1916, one month after she had written the antisuffrage, anti–birth control letter to the *New York Post,* Putnam received a letter from the newly founded Birth Control League of Massachusetts (BCLM). The letter asked her to take a seat on the platform at two mass birth control meetings at the Majestic and Globe Theaters. The BCLM's tone is reminiscent of the deferential treatment Putnam received by staff of the CB in this same period. In addition to asking her to take a prominent position at their mass meetings, another letter added that the League, "should be genuinely grateful if you could find the time to suggest better ways of education than we are using to promote this movement, the only handicap of which seems to be the ignorance of the populace."[59]

The BCLM was clearly trying to strengthen its cause through affiliation with reputable citizens. Charles Zeublin of the BCLM ostensibly expected support from Putnam because of her involvement in what he considered the complementary field of prenatal care. However, in his letter, he tried to appeal to her patriotism. Putnam was a member of the Special Aid Society for American Preparedness and, therefore, he reasoned that she "must believe in the desirability of reducing the number of unfit citizens."[60] He chose to represent his group's goal as the "demand that mothers shall choose the time of the birth of future American citizens."[61] Although Putnam was a zealous patriot, it seems clear that Zeublin would have had more luck engaging her sympathies if he had addressed Putnam as an expert and pioneer in the prenatal care movement. In this period her ties with the AASPIM and the CB were still strong. Zeublin might have done better to mention her knowledge of the suffering of women in childbirth, or the problems associated with frequent and unhealthy pregnancies for both mothers and infants. But, on the contrary, he attempted to cloak the aim of the BCLM in patriotic language that did not necessarily have the same power as an appeal to Putnam's consciousness of herself as an innovator in maternal health care. Zeublin's correspondence with Putnam shows the extent to which the members of the BCLM were themselves intimidated by the radical implications of their cause and the extent to which they sought to broaden their coalition of support. This issue will be examined further in chapter 4.

Putnam responded to the inquiries of the BCLM in an ambivalent manner. Although she stated clearly that she was opposed to birth control, she admitted a great interest in the issue and asked for literature: "I certainly agree with you as to the desirability—or rather the necessity—of reducing the number of births of unfit citizens, but I do not believe in the methods of the Birth Control League for accomplishing this result, and, therefore, I must, with many thanks for your courtesy, decline to sit on the platform on October first. I think your objects can be met better in other ways . . .—but as I am greatly interested in the subject, I should be glad to see your literature if you will kindly send it to me."[62] Thus, Putnam, did not want to be cut off completely from the birth control movement. Her desire for their literature as well as the BCLM's requests for her coopera- tion attests to an acknowledged commonality among reproductive reformers.

In the following spring the BCLM again tried to coax Putnam into its ranks. Mary East, secretary of the BCLM, tried a different tactic to make her appeal for support:

> Believing that you have a genuine interest in matters which concern the physical welfare of our people and the economic prosperity of our country, I am taking the liberty of writing you concerning the Massachusetts Birth Control League. In common with the leading sociologists of to-day, we feel that a real menace exists in the present reckless increase of children condemned to poverty, ignorance and neglect, while at the same time the birth rate among those who have risen through better hereditary endow- ments continues to decline. Intelligent and voluntary motherhood has taken the place of heedless and immoral propagation among the educated classes, it is right that it should.[63]

The League preferred to define its efforts as eugenic, patriotic, and med- ically and monetarily sound. As a subsequent chapter will show, these tac- tics revealed an ambivalence about the radical implication of the cause as well as a desire to be associated with social welfare.

The next opportunity the Massachusetts birth control reformers had for recruiting Putnam to their ranks came when they officially reorga- nized their organization as the Family Welfare Foundation in the sum- mer of 1919. This change was predicated on the assumption that the movement could attract greater numbers if it lost its association with the radicalism of Margaret Sanger and the national movement. The new name served to cloak advocacy of birth control as yet another pro-family reform effort. Putnam was precisely the kind of person the birth con- trollers hoped to attract with this political strategy. She committed her- self to improving the lives of mothers and children and therefore, the Family Welfare Foundation believed she would undoubtedly appreciate the need for family planning for at least eugenic, medical, or economic reasons.

In July 1919 Putnam received a letter from Vera P. Lane of the Fam- ily Welfare Foundation announcing the change in its name. Lane explained that, along with the name, the old group had changed and reorganized along a broader, more constructive policy. She went on to ask Putnam to become a member and to contribute money. Less than one week later, Lane sent Putnam a more personalized letter in which she specifically addressed Putnam's previously stated position on birth control: "I note your letter in the files of April 28, 1917 and find that you are in sympathy as to the desirability of limiting undesirable births, but do not approve of the methods of the League. . . . There were many members of the old league who agreed with you as to methods, myself included. . . . If you are willing to give me a half hour some day very soon, I would like to talk with you in detail about the plans for new work.[64]

The Massachusetts reformers were not the only birth control reformers attempting to recruit Putnam in this period. Mary Ware Dennett also tried to encourage Putnam to support her legislative efforts by stressing her "public health and welfare" background:

> Several groups of reputable citizens who have public health and welfare at heart, are now being invited to sign the enclosed endorsement which will be presented to Congress when our measure is introduced at the winter session. . . . If you picture how it will increase the health and happiness when physicians, clinics, dispensaries, hospitals and the various health agencies are free to give this much needed information on sex hygiene, you will, I am sure, be glad to add your name to the daily increasing list of distinguished people who endorse our primary aim.[65]

Putnam never responded to Dennett's appeal. While she responded to fellow middle- and upper-class Boston female reformers, if even to politely decline an offer to become involved in the Family Welfare Foundation, Putnam had no ties to birth control reformers such as Dennett.

Putnam's refusal to associate herself with the birth control movement reflected and reinforced her ideological ties with the majority of maternal and infant health care reformers in this period. Both Putnam and the women in the CB resisted this more individualistic and controversial solution to the problem of infant and maternal mortality. However, this agreement over birth control did not form the basis of a lasting coalition between Putnam and the women in the CB. While members of the CB shied away from associations with radicalism for political or expedient reasons, Putnam reacted to the solution of birth control like many nineteenth-century women reformers in her abhorrence of its potential to separate the act of sex from procreation. But Putnam's reluctance to accept birth control as a legitimate strategy for social reform was neither steadfast nor simple. By the late 1920s, as we shall see, the evolution of her political agenda would once again bring back the issue of birth control for her consideration.

CHOOSING SIDES: THE POLITICS OF SHEPPARD-TOWNER

The origins of the strain in relations between Putnam and the staff of the CB can be found in the late teens when the Bureau began working toward the passage of a federal maternity and infancy bill. This project marked the beginning of the brief second phase of Putnam's reform career. A simultaneous development that discouraged continued amiability between Putnam and the women in the CB was Putnam's rising status in the Republican Party. In 1920 she became the first woman elected president of an electoral college in Massachusetts. In 1923 she was the first woman to run for delegate-at-large to the Republican National Convention. That same year she was elected president of the Coolidge Women's Clubs of America. Putnam vigorously supported Coolidge's campaign for the presidency in 1924.

In 1920 Putnam had actively campaigned for the Massachusetts Maternity and Infancy Bill. However, her enthusiasm did not extend to the national bill sponsored by the CB and supported by the General Federation of Women's Clubs. Only six months after she played a vital role in securing the passage of a statewide maternal health care measure, she wrote to Senator Henry Cabot Lodge to voice her opposition to the Sheppard-Towner Bill.

> I am very sorry to see that this bill passed the Senate, because it seems to me a very seriously objectionable measure in that it puts the control of the care of child birth under the Secretary of Labor and the head of the CB, who naturally has no knowledge of medicine . . . The head of the CB, through her "Children's Year" campaign, roused the unthinking women of the country to think more of their children's health. It was a good deed, but it has not made the women of the country capable of deciding who is the best fitted person to supervise the health of themselves and their children. Obviously it is not the Secretary of Labor, and equally obviously the executive officer of maternity care should not be a lay woman. There is just one body in the country who ought to be put in charge of this work and of all the health work throughout the United States, and that is the Department of Public Health.[66]

It is clear from this letter that, at this point in 1921, Putnam's objections to Sheppard-Towner were reasonable and well considered. She did not yet exhibit an irrational fear of communism that would plague her in the years immediately before her death. Nor did she voice a comprehensive hatred of the CB. In this second phase of her reform career, she simply argued that the administration of Sheppard-Towner was in the wrong hands.

Putnam's objections to the Sheppard-Towner Bill were seconded by other reputable people and organizations in the infant welfare movement. The U.S. Public Health Service, for example, sought jurisdiction over questions of maternity and infancy, and resented the power granted to an organization within the Department of Labor. Similarly, the American Child Hygiene Association (ACHA)—which Putnam was still affiliated with—approved of the purpose of the bill, but disapproved of some of its methods. Dr. S. Josephine Baker, president of the ACHA and head of the innovative New York City Bureau of Child Hygiene, argued at legislative hearings in 1919 that the Sheppard-Towner Bill threatened the autonomy of local boards of health already in existence by seeking to establish state boards of maternal and infant welfare.[67] Like Putnam, Baker objected both to the unnecessary expansion of bureaucracy and the amount of power these centralizing efforts would give the federal government over local agencies.[68] The ACHA had been involved in establishing divisions of child hygiene on the state and municipal levels since its formation in 1909. Although the ACHA supported the establishment of both the CB and a federal department of health, it was wary of both duplication and usurpation of effort.

Five months after writing her initial letter of opposition to Senator Lodge, Putnam wrote to Lodge again and "enclosed . . . a copy of the Sheppard-Towner Bill with the amendments which would in our (our refers to ACHA) opinion make it a proper bill to pass."[69] In this letter, Putnam changed her tactic a bit and first began to object to what she called the federal government's paternalism. However, she did not yet reject outright the federal government's authority in the field of maternal and infant health. She specifically opposed setting up a structure that would subject state medical authorities to the "approval of the social worker at the head of the CB in Washington."[70] Putnam wrote to Lodge:

> If . . . Congress decides that this is a matter for federal control, I believe that it should be put under the Public Health Service rather than the CB. . . . The CB was formed in 1912 to investigate and report on matters concerning children. It was given no administrative power beyond the publication of its

reports, and its functions have never been increased by Congress. Should it undertake the care of maternity it would enter into and usurp the work of another division of government, namely, the Public Health Service.[71]

CB officials denied the charge that their work duplicated that of the Public Health Service (PHS). They contended that any health plan must, to be successful, go beyond strictly medical provisions to deal with social and environmental factors. Because of their holistic philosophy, they rejected the more narrowly conventional medical approach of the PHS as inadequate to deal with the complex issues surrounding maternal and infant mortality, and resisted attempts to be taken over by medical authorities.[72]

Putnam also opposed what she regarded as Sheppard-Towner's emphasis on education at the expense of medical treatment. She argued that, "You cannot instruct an expectant mother how to overcome pelvic abnormalities, prevent post-partum hemorrhage, to prevent infection at the hands of poorly trained nurses, midwives, and physicians. . . . It is ignorance that causes deaths in maternity and early infancy, but it is not education that the mother needs to prevent it, except insofar as she needs to be educated that care of maternity is a medical matter. . . . Prenatal care can never be given by education."[73] Putnam's willingness to define prenatal care as a purely medical issue certainly marked a shift in her perspective, one that coincided with the CB's change of leadership and its attempt to significantly enlarge its sphere of authority. Both of these factors influenced Putnam's censure. While Putnam at one time harbored great respect for Julia Lathrop, she disliked Grace Abbott and resented the power that the passage of Sheppard-Towner would grant her.

The American Medical Association (AMA) shared Putnam's two major concerns over Sheppard-Towner, namely, that it would usurp the authority of physicians and local boards of health, and that it was to be administered by the wrong federal department. Putnam had always maintained a good relationship with the organized medical community by acknowledging its crucial role in improving prenatal care. In 1921, Putnam published a letter in the *Journal of the American Medical Association* (*JAMA*) opposing Sheppard-Towner, but when Grace Abbott sought to present her side of the case in the journal, she was told that the issue was not relevant to *JAMA* readers.[74] Yet Putnam's attitude toward the AMA and the medical community was not entirely uncritical. For example, earlier she had warned physicians that it would be difficult to "crowd out" the midwives if medical schools did not begin to pay more attention to obstetrics and gynecology.[75]

Putnam based her outspoken critique of Sheppard-Towner on her expertise in the field of infant and maternal health care. She assured Lodge in 1921 that "in opposing this bill I am doing it only for the welfare of the women and children, for which object I have worked for the last twelve years."[76] By 1921, Dr. S. Josephine Baker of the ACHA had come to approve of the final version of the Sheppard-Towner Bill. Putnam not only disagreed with Baker but was disgruntled that Baker had been treated by Congress and the press as the principal authority in this field. After reading the Congressional records of the Sheppard-Towner hearings, Putnam charged that Baker was, "quoted as the authority all through the speeches in the House made in favor of the bill, because she is apparently considered the pioneer in the subject, when she not only was not the pioneer but is barking up the wrong tree in my opinion, in supporting this bill."[77] Putnam went on to add that Baker was very capable and a great friend of hers, but that she simply was making an incorrect judgment in supporting the Sheppard-Towner Bill.

The year that Sheppard-Towner was passed, Putnam was one of its most outspoken critics. However, she continually expressed the need for some type of legislative action in regard to maternal and infant health care. Her primary motive in the second period of her reform career continued to be the health of mothers and children. She had not yet disavowed the need for a federal CB, nor had she completely ruled out the notion that some version of the federal maternity and infancy bill could be helpful. In a letter to the *JAMA*, Putnam admitted that the Sheppard-Towner plan would surely save some lives, but not as many as would be possible if its methods were reconsidered. She wrote, "The bill will do good. Almost any bill bearing on the subject, administered in any way, is sure to do good, because the conditions are now so very bad that almost any plan can hardly fail to improve them—but must we stop at an inferior thing?"[78]

Putnam's disapproval of the Sheppard-Towner plan went hand in hand with her dislike and mistrust of Grace Abbott. Putnam did not believe that Abbott could compare to Lathrop in terms of her abilities, and made her feelings known quite publicly in speeches.[79]

One of the issues that served to alienate Putnam and Abbott was the midwife question. In 1924 a bill was introduced in the Massachusetts legislature to legalize and license the practice of midwifery. Putnam took a strong stand against this bill, arguing, "The laws regarding the practice of medicine in this state are already disgracefully lax. Do not let us relax them further at the expense of the poor. Let us rather devote ourselves to raising the standards of medicine."[80] Here Putnam was echoing a mainstream viewpoint in reproductive reform circles. In 1911, for example, obstetrician and AASPIM board member J. Whitridge Williams delivered an influential address in which he argued "that the remedy for the low level of obstetrical care in American lay not in licensing and legitimizing female midwifery, but in improving the skill of doctors."[81]

Abbott supported legalization and licensing of midwives. According to CB historian Kristin Lindenmeyer, "Abbott conceded that it was, at least for the time being, inevitable that some women would use midwives. Therefore, under Sheppard-Towner, the CB encouraged states to develop midwife training programs and enforce (or establish) state licensing."[82] Thus, while obstetrical care was still unavailable to countless women, Abbott "conceded the economic and cultural necessity of midwives."[83] Putnam ridiculed Abbott's position on midwifery as amounting to ignorance and disregard for women's lives. In a letter to the *Independent,* Putnam claimed that Abbott had once told her "that her mother was delivered of her by a midwife and what was good enough for her mother was good enough for anyone." She added, "This is the woman in whose hands the Government has put the welfare of the children of the country and through the Sheppard-Towner act the welfare of women in childbirth."[84]

By the end of the second phase of Putnam's career, it was clear that she stood apart from what had now become the "mainstream" of maternal and child welfare reformers. While the CB and its allies promoted programs of their own creation, Putnam endorsed a more conventionally medical, doctor-centered approach to maternal and child health. Adamant in her beliefs, Putnam attempted to impede the growth of any type of program that embodied the values she rejected. This objective meshed nicely with her conservative opposition to any expansion of the federal government (except for the medically dominated Public Health Service), and pitted her squarely against the "female dominion."

No Prisoners: Putnam Takes on the CB

By the mid-1920s Putnam's critique of Sheppard-Towner developed into a full-fledged attack on the CB. This shift marked the third stage in Putnam's career when her conservative politics brought her into direct conflict with the reproductive health mainstream. Whereas she had once been a proud supporter of the work of the CB, Putnam now vigorously opposed it.

This conflict came to a head in 1927, when Sheppard-Towner was originally scheduled to expire, but debates opened to extend its appropriation. Putnam's objections to the extension of Sheppard-Towner for even one more day blossomed into overall opposition to federal attention to matters of maternity, and the mere existence of the U. S. Children's Bureau. Voicing some of her objections to William Graham of the House of Representatives, she requested a Congressional investigation of the Bureau: "The CB is an objectionable thing, full of fads and undigested theories, costing the country much money annually and eager to cost it still more. Could not an impartial investigation of it be undertaken, which would bring to light much that the public ought to know? Of course I am aware that it is entrenched in the hearts of masses of unthinking women, such as the Federated Women's Clubs, etc., but I believe these women could be convinced by facts if they were properly presented to them."[85] The unthinking women to whom Putnam alluded also became increasing targets of her belligerence in the late 1920s and early 1930s. While years before she had attempted to forge and keep cordial relations with the GFWC in her efforts to pass milk legislation and spread the word about prenatal care, she now referred to them derisively as "the emotional mob-ridden organization women."[86]

From the late 1920s until her death in 1935, Putnam did not relax her efforts to publicly discredit the CB. In a letter to the *American Journal of Obstetrics and Gynecology* in 1929, Putnam wrote, "The more statistics they roll up, the more anyone can see how absolutely nothing they have accomplished."[87] In a speech delivered in 1930 entitled "Decentralization versus Patriotism," Putnam used spurious logic to debunk the CB. She argued that "Contagious diseases . . . are a matter for protection by the federal government, but matters like the care of maternity and infancy have no concern with it whatever—maternity has never been considered a contagious disease—hence the CB is an utterly unnecessary body."[88] Putnam adeptly combined her accusations of ineffectuality with fiscal conservatism when she wrote: "Infant mortality is lower among states which have not accepted the Sheppard-Towner Act than among those who have. . . . This seems hardly worth spending a million and a quarter dollars to accomplish! It seems rather tough to exact taxes from the citizens of the U.S. to support a lot of employees who are so incompetent."[89]

In addition to citing its ineptitude and cost, Putnam became obsessed with the notion that the CB was connected to the threat of international communism. In a speech before the Daughters of 1812, Putnam commended the following resolution on the CB made by the conservative women's group: "The only justification for such Bureaucratic supervision of homes and children is in a communist state. In the U.S. the very existence of such a bureau is an insult to American parents."[90] Putnam then urged her audience to act upon their resolution.

Grace Abbott continued to be a particular target of Putnam's. Now, however, Putnam not only accused her of incompetence and ignorance, but also claimed, on the basis of personal knowledge, that Abbott was "directly under the Soviet government."[91] Conveniently forgetting her earlier affiliation and support of its work, Putnam now argued that, "The creation of the CB in the Department of Labor in Washington was the first subversive achievement over American Government and Institutions, and the earliest Communist foothold in the Federal Government, obtained by Florence Kelley . . . disciple and translator of Friedrich Engels."[92] Putnam exaggerated Kelley's influence in the CB and the federal government, while almost never mentioning the significant role played by Lathrop or West in shaping the agenda of the CB. Likewise, Putnam never referred to her own enthusiastic support of the CB and her efforts to help them with their publications and with obtaining adequate funding in the early years. On the contrary, Putnam now argued that, "The CB was established in 1912 not in response to popular demand, for self-reliant, resourceful and energetic American parents never dreamed of Bureaus in 130 years of American democracy. But, influenced by Mrs. Kelley and others who conducted a seven year propaganda campaign, led Congress to impose it upon the American people."[93]

Putnam's involvement with the Sentinels of the Republic (established in 1922) illustrates the extent to which a commitment to curb the growth of the federal government overwhelmed other social and political concerns by the end of her life. She became a member of the Boston Committee of the Sentinels in 1926. The Sentinels strictly adhered to the principle of limited government and strove to fulfill the following purposes: to maintain the fundamental principles of the Constitution, to oppose further federal encroachment on state and individual rights, to stop the spread of Communism, to stop the expansion of bureaucracy, and to preserve the republican form of government in the United States. Under the list of its achievements and successes, the Sentinels took at least some credit for defeating the Child Labor Amendment, the repeal of Sheppard-Towner, and the opposition to the creation of a federal Department of Education.[94] Among the groups it opposed were some with which Putnam once had amicable relations, including the General Federation of Women's Clubs, the American Child Health Association, and the Children's Bureau. Other groups considered threats had long been on Putnam's list of enemies, including the National League of Women Voters, National Council of Women, National Women's Party, and the National Women's Trade Union League. The Sentinels both shaped and validated the further entrenchment of Putnam's political views.

Although she herself precipitated her own separation from the larger reform community, Putnam never seemed comfortable with the drop in status and power this separation necessarily demanded. Indeed, she blamed mainstream reformers for slighting her record of achievements and pushing her out of power. Interpreting the course of events that led to her resignation and alienation from the ACHA, for example, Putnam had this to say to A. Piatt Andrew: "Mr. Hoover is too closely associated with the people of the Child Health Organization of which I was president during the war and who afterwards got in such close cahoots with the CB that they kicked me off the executive committee in order to keep Grace Abbott on and they have made Mr. Hoover their first continuous president. . . . They have slighted me nobly."[95] To Dr. Tagliaferro Clark of the U.S. Public Health Service, she wrote: "I am too blunt and hot tempered to be popular, unfortunately. There are those who love and respect me but very few, I am afraid, who like me."[96] The bitterness evident in Putnam's description of her experience with the people in the ACHA can be found throughout her personal correspondence in the late 1920s. In an unusually revealing and vulnerable moment Putnam wrote, "You know I made the initial experiment in the world on the value of prenatal care. . . . But I am better known in Australia than in my own land and city. It is a funny world, isn't it? Sometimes a bit heart-breaking."[97]

As Putnam became increasingly alienated from mainstream reproductive reformers, she drifted closer not only toward conservative groups like the Sentinels, but to the organized and powerful medical community. This alliance was founded on a mutual opposition to the laywomen in the Department of Labor who were purportedly trying to control America's children and usurp the proper role of physicians. Once Putnam had cut her ties with both the ACHA and the CB, she found a receptive audience in the AMA and the Public Health Service. In addition to Dr. Tagliaferro Clark, Putnam found an ally in Dr. George Kosmak, the editor of the *American Journal of Obstetrics and Gynecology*. She confided in them and encouraged them to lead the fight against the CB and the reinstatement of Sheppard-Towner-type legislation. In October, 1929 Putnam asked Dr. Clark, "Would the Public Health Service undertake anything in obstetrics—and if not, why not?"[98] She informed him that she had already written to the previous president of the AMA "to suggest that doctors need to take up this reform so as to forestall the CB's efforts to reinstate Sheppard-Towner."[99] Earlier that year, Putnam wrote to Dr. Kosmak and asked if he "could not persuade the AMA to take hold of the teaching of obstetrics throughout the medical schools of the country and set a standard for the medical schools in that respect, as they have in so many others . . . ?"[100] She also suggested that the AMA agitate for changes in the medical school curriculum so as to emphasize and further professionalize the field of obstetrics.

Since 1909, when she began her prenatal care experiment, Putnam had recognized the need for upgrading medical research, training, and care for women and children. Her conservative politics enabled her to envision free and unregulated professionals striving to improve their services to individuals, but no longer to see the benefit of governmental regulation or intervention. In contrast to her colleagues in the CB, Putnam had come to view prenatal care strictly as a medical issue. Indeed, Putnam's insistence that social conditions were basically irrelevant to maternal and infant mortality defied the results of the groundbreaking local studies undertaken by the CB.

In the fall of 1929 Putnam began working on a new scheme to undermine the CB. She stopped trying to convince more liberal reformers to submit to her way of thinking, and instead planned to organize a group of conservative women into political action. She first referred to her plan in a letter to Dr. Clark in October 1929: "Whereas the Federated Women's Clubs are behind the CB, there is a much larger number of women outside of the Federated Women's Clubs who are sane thinking and would be behind a sound movement—especially one inaugurated for protection of women and children in childbirth."[101] Putnam imagined that this alternative movement to protect women and children in childbirth would be led by the medical profession, either through the U.S. Public Health Service or through the AMA. Putnam assured Clark that she had already been approached by a friend who asked for help in starting a group of "sane—though often silent—women of the country who far outnumber the noisy ones now collected together in clubs."[102]

Mrs. Francis E. Slattery approached Putnam in 1929 and together in 1930 they formed the Women's National League to Protect Our Homes and Children. Slattery was the arch-conservative head of the League of Catholic Women in Massachusetts and a member of the executive committee of the Sentinels of the Republic. Originally, Putnam described the new organization as a "nation wide organization of women for the Maintenance of the Duties and Privileges of the States under the Federal Constitution."[103] This description underscores Putnam's growing commitment to curbing the role of the federal government. Whereas she had originally entered political life in order to improve maternal and infant health care, her new political goals revolved around loyalty to a platform of fiscal conservatism, states' rights, and anticommunism. Reproductive health reform receded from her agenda, as its promotion now seemed inextricably bound up with federal programs she distrusted.

Putnam's curious political trajectory from quasi-progressive to arch-conservative can be partially explained by particular political circumstances in Massachusetts. By the 1920s, the state's progressive coalition had been torn apart by inter-ethnic and religious suspicion and enmity. Old-stock Americans' call for educational reform, prohibition, and other measures considered by newer Catholic immigrants to be attempts at Americanization led to the latter group's defection from the reform ranks and "suspicion of reform in general."[104] Once the ethnic cooperation that was vital to the success of Massachusetts's progressivism was lost, the conservatives—consisting of newer U.S. Catholics and economic conservatives—gained control of the state. The growth of this powerful coalition attracted the likes of Putnam and facilitated her steering away from her earlier commitments. This same political climate also made the struggle for birth control an especially arduous one in Massachusetts, as chapter 4 will show.

As active members of the Sentinels, Putnam and Slattery quite naturally opposed President Herbert Hoover's amicable relations with the CB and his growing acceptance of federal solutions for the country's economic troubles. The two women sought an audience with President Hoover to discuss their concerns. On March 3, 1930, Slattery and Putnam had a generally unsuccessful yet highly publicized meeting with President Hoover. They explained to Hoover that the CB was "being run by a bunch of Communists."[105] Slattery and Putnam told Hoover that they were opposed to the "nationalization" of American's children through the centralized power of the CB, and warned that the nation's families would not tolerate another maternity act similar in scope to the now-expired Sheppard-Towner. They also expressed their support of states' rights and a small federal budget. An article from the *Boston Herald* summed up their agenda in one concise sentence: "Besides pointing to the increase in the maternal death rate since the operation of the act, its opponents also say that it is a step toward federal bureaucracy, an invasion of states' right and a scheme to make jobs for welfare workers."[106]

In this last stage of Putnam's political career, which was characterized by movement away from the female dominion and its reproductive health agenda, she began to reconsider the issue of birth control. While birth control may have been anathema to Putnam's Victorian conception of sexuality, it could fit neatly with her political ideology. Once the larger maternal and infant welfare movement became synonymous with movements to increase federal intervention in the family, Putnam began to consider the merits of birth control as a possible way around this correlation. In other words, Putnam's antistate posture and her faith in medicine led her to explore new avenues of reform that would have otherwise continued to repel her. This surprising turn underscores both the interconnectedness of reproductive reform issues, and the impact of political circumstances on their fate.

In 1927 Putnam wrote to Dr. Robert L. Dickinson in order to obtain reliable information on birth control. Dickinson had been the executive secretary of the Committee on Maternal Health in New York City, and the president of the American Gynecological Society. He supported birth control and had worked with Margaret Sanger on her legislative reform campaigns. She sought statistics from Dickinson on the various methods of birth control and their reliability. Putnam's decision to contact Dickinson, rather than Sanger, Dennett, or Ames, reflected her shift away from the women's reform community. Putnam identified herself to Dickinson by writing, "I am the Mrs. Putnam who made the initial experiment in the value of prenatal care and I have for the past eighteen years been very much interested in all that concerning the subject of maternity and infancy."[107] Thus, by 1927, Putnam articulated the connection between her own work and the goals of the birth control movement—the very point birth control activists had been trying to make ten years earlier.

Putnam showed other signs that her conservative political orientation could potentially bring her closer to reproductive rights, as she began to take up the related issue of censorship. In a speech before the Parliamentary Law Club in April 1927, Putnam thoroughly chided Anthony Comstock and his censorship authority in a manner that would have made the most fervent birth controller proud: "Only one who is omniscient can properly be a censor and the willingness to undertake the task indicates an assumption of omniscience which argues an almost complete state of ignorance, because the more knowledge one possesses the more clearly one sees the limitless bounds of what one does not know."[108] Putnam did not necessarily have birth control in mind when she objected to the Comstock censorship laws. However, Comstock was indelibly linked in the public mind with social purity campaigns. In fact, Putnam added some levity to her address by charging that Comstock would be likely to order skirts on Greek statues.[109]

Putnam's anticensorship stance surfaced just as her position against prohibition became more clearly defined. She simply did not believe that the federal government had a right to intervene into private life, whether through censorship or prohibition. While many old-stock Americans in the Republican Party remained committed to the Eighteenth Amendment, Putnam joined the Women's Organization for National Prohibition Reform in 1929. Echoing her opposition to legislation such as

Sheppard-Towner, Putnam argued, "Prohibition cannot be a matter of national legislation, for it is a sumptuary law, and sumptuary laws are not a matter for the federal government to take up."[110] Putnam defined her position as pro-temperance but anti-Prohibition in order to distinguish her personal, moral beliefs from her sense of an appropriate role for federal government. This distinction between Putnam's personal commitments and her political agenda also entered her maternalist politics. Although committed to transforming and improving prenatal care services available to U.S. women, Putnam increasingly looked toward the medical profession and private enterprise to achieve this goal. As birth control could fit more neatly with this political orientation than with social services, Putnam's interest in the former issue was peaked. In fact, in 1930 Putnam put off her friend Slattery's suggestion that she engage herself in the battle against birth control. Slattery's leadership position in the League of Catholic Women virtually assured her rejection of birth control. However, Putnam demurred, citing extremism on both sides of the issue.[111]

CONCLUSION

Putnam's career shows that there was certainly no one way that middle-class and elite white women welfare reformers viewed the meaning of state responsibility and power, nor was there agreement on the most efficient and humane way of aiding mothers and children. Although an innovator in the field and a temporary ally, Putnam's world view and background were decidedly different from the majority of reproductive health activists. Putnam had no training in the social sciences and no experience with the settlement house movement beyond a superficial affiliation in the prewar years with the South End House and the Cambridge Neighborhood House. Kathryn Kish Sklar has argued that social science in the early twentieth century, especially the nonacademic social science practiced by female reformers, embraced as its principal mission the expansion of the federal government into an active protector of its most vulnerable citizens.[112] For the majority of reproductive health reformers, therefore, the task of improving the conditions of maternity and infancy went hand in hand with expanding the role of the state.

Another basic difference between Putnam and the majority of her colleagues in the reproductive health movement was Putnam's failure to connect the vulnerability of mothers and children with the vulnerability of other members of society. Progressive maternalists fought not only to protect women and children through government intervention, but also immigrants and laborers. Their social justice ideals developed in the Progressive Era and carried them through to support the innovations of the New Deal.

In addition to highlighting diversity among reproductive reformers, Putnam's career illustrates the impact of political circumstances on their agendas. Her fear of federal paternalism represented a powerful political force in the interwar years and helps to explain why the maternalist coalition began to falter. As reproductive health activism became synonymous with federal activism, Putnam's commitment to states' rights and a small federal role encouraged her flight from this cohort. As politics caused rifts, it also made strange bedfellows, as we have seen in the example of Putnam's reconsideration of birth control. Ironically, birth control could provide this conservative reformer with a way to continue her crusade to aid mothers and children while avoiding the pitfalls of centralization and bureaucratization.

Finally, Putnam provides a lens through which to evaluate the work of the CB during the era of their triumph and decline, underscoring the Bureau's widespread attraction to maternalists across the political spectrum in its early years; its consistent devotion to the disadvantaged; and its failure to transcend political debates over the role of the state by the late 1920s.

2

"The whole problem of motherhood"

ETHEL STURGES DUMMER, FEMINISM

DELINQUENCY, AND ILLEGITIMACY

Whereas Elizabeth Putnam's conservative politics facilitated her volatile rift with the female dominion, Ethel Dummer's feminism spurred frustration and an ultimately more amicable break. Along the spectrum of concern for the welfare of mothers and children, Ethel Sturges Dummer was unique in her unapologetic advocacy of women's emancipation, her critique of conventional morality, and her dedication to vulnerable citizens. In 1920 she wrote about the swirling discourses that surrounded and bolstered her in her search for equality and social justice: "Creative energy is simply sweeping away the wrongs of women, which have long been ignored. . . . The subject grows complex. One group cries *mutterschutz,* another birth control, while echoes of divorce, mother-endowment, elimination of prostitution, psychoanalysis reach our ears."[1] As this quote illustrates, Dummer possessed an optimistic spirit that was nurtured by her willingness to see many avenues available to those who sought to improve maternal welfare. While Putnam came to reproductive reform through her interest in saving the lives of babies and mothers, and that medical orientation remained the fulcrum of her politics, Dummer came to reproductive reform through a very different route—one that began with redressing wrongs done to women and moved her towards vulnerable and disadvantaged mothers. Incorporating reproductive health and reproductive rights issues, Dummer's orientation is perhaps the broadest of all of the four women in this study. She rejected nothing that she believed might bring the desired results. This trait was both her greatest strength as a theorist, and her greatest weakness as a political activist.

Dummer came to reproductive reform via a circuitous route that began with her patronage of the Chicago Juvenile Court (which reflected an interest in female delinquency) and led ultimately to a radical perspective on motherhood, sexuality, and illegitimacy. She was a philanthropist who possessed the spirit of an insurgent. Her wealth allowed her to fund projects and individuals that promised to bring the social and political changes for which she strove. According to sociologist Jennifer Platt, Dummer's "preferred mode of action was to be the means by which others carried out what she thought was needed. However, to see this as the natural mode of operation for a wealthy woman who had nothing to offer but her money and her social contacts would be highly misleading about the nature of her contribution."[2] Indeed, Dummer was more than a patron or philanthropist, as she herself engaged in and encouraged innovative research in the social sciences. She made a career of discovering and supporting "cutting-edge" people and projects, and then disseminating their work throughout progressive reform circles. Dummer herself characterized her unique efforts as "acting as a switchboard, connecting people and ideas."[3] In contrast to Putnam, she did not seek leadership positions or engage in self-promotion. Therefore, her reform career took on a very different shape in terms of both strategies and goals.

This chapter will examine Dummer's political activities in the arena of reproductive reform from the prewar years through the 1930s. During these decades, even as her feminism brought her into conflict with the mainstream reform community, she funded projects in the social sciences and social welfare arena that were among the most significant of the era. She served on the Illinois Juvenile Protection Agency (JPA); was a member of the Committee on Protective Work for Girls during World War I; was a patron of the Chicago Juvenile Court; founded and was a trustee of the Chicago School for Civics and Philanthropy; launched an experimental visiting obstetrical nurse program upon which Sheppard-Towner was based; and worked tirelessly to improve the treatment of unwed mothers.

Dummer's reproductive reform activities provide an important counterpoint to both Putnam and the Children's Bureau (CB) in terms of the causes she championed and the political perspective she embodied. While Putnam came to represent a larger group of conservative reformers who sought to undermine the progressive social welfare agenda of agencies like the CB, Dummer sought to advance the goals of feminists and radical social reformers. According to Wendy Sarvasy, the aim of the latter groups was nothing less than "to transform gender relations and women's values through the creation of a feminist, not a maternalist, welfare state."[4] Thus,

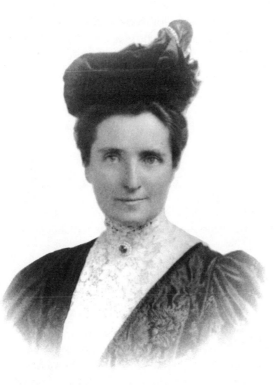

FIG. 2 ETHEL STURGES DUMMER.
Photo courtesy of the Schlesinger Library, Radcliffe
Institute, Harvard University.

Dummer's career in reproductive reform offers a decisive contrast to both the CB's maternalism and Putnam's antistatism.

While the thrust of Putnam's orientation and activism illustrates by way of contrast the CB's dedication to the poor, Dummer's direction reveals a certain degree of timidity in the Bureau's agenda in contrast to her own commitment to broad social and cultural change. Indeed, Dummer's career exposes four significant and interconnected tendencies of the CB: neglecting the reproductive rights of women, ignoring the nonprocreative aspects of female sexuality, utilizing policy to shore up the traditional family, and, finally, recognizing women's needs only as they emanate from their maternal responsibilities. However, Dummer's contrasting career also reflects the tenacity of the CB in the face of the hostile political climate of the 1920s. While Dummer embraced more radical and certainly more feminist goals than her counterparts in the Bureau, she ultimately became disenchanted with social policy and shifted toward the more apolitical field of psychology. Dummer's radicalism led her to "burn out" and leave the fray while administrators in the CB held fast to their social welfare agenda. Thus, Dummer presents an interesting foil to the Bureau as she exposes both its limits and its impressive resolve during the difficult interwar years.

∞

Dummer was born into a wealthy Chicago family, the third of nine children of George and Mary (Delafield) Sturges. The daughter of a bank president, Ethel married the vice president of her father's bank in 1888. Her husband, William Francis Dummer, also belonged to a distinguished Massachusetts family and took an interest in civics, social reform, and politics. Ethel Dummer was herself a firm believer in *noblesse oblige,* schooled at the Kirkland School by such reform-minded women as Ellen Gates Starr, cofounder of Hull House. Indeed, she was to spend the greater part of her adult life generating and sustaining various political and intellectual projects through financial contributions and her personal efforts.

The Dummers had five children, four of whom, all daughters, survived into adulthood. The experience of an infant death was one that Ethel shared with both Elizabeth Putnam and Mary Dennett, and indeed with many women in this period. Although they never expressed it publicly, it would be naïve to think that that the subsequent dedication these women exhibited in various movements to improve the health and welfare of mothers and children was not in some way connected to their tragic personal experiences.[5] However, the paths they chose reflected their political orientations as much as their individual circumstances and stories.

Dummer's reform career began like that of so many other middle-class and wealthy white women in Progressive-Era Chicago: with an interest in the problem of child labor. She considered this cause to be her political awakening, acknowledging that her privileged position might have easily shielded her from the wider world. In her autobiography she wrote, "Surely in my generation there were many blinded by the sunshine of their own lives to the shadows of others."[6] Literature from the National Child Labor Committee (NCLC) led Dummer to a conference, where she heard Jane Addams and Felix Frankfurter speak on this issue. She recalled years later that this event began a new epoch for herself and her husband, as her "social conscience was born."[7] Whereas Putnam fought child labor reform as an unwanted intrusion into family life in these same years, Dummer embraced this movement as the instigator of her political awakening. Indeed, Dummer's involvement in the issue of child labor nurtured a rich social conscience and lifelong sense of social and political responsibility to the less fortunate.

Child labor led Dummer to a more general interest in the welfare of children and the burgeoning fields of social work and sociology. She quickly joined both the NCLC and the JPA and immersed herself in the "sins and sufferings of humanity."[8] Had Dummer's temperament been different, the world she was exposed to through her work with the JPA could have brought an untimely end to her career as a reformer and philanthropist. Instead of shying away from the sordid nature of this work, Dummer forged ahead and, through an association with Hull House and the University of Chicago Settlement, became even more involved with direct social services to troubled and needy children. It was at this time in her life that Dummer acknowledged a shift in her perspective "from philanthropy to civics."[9] By this claim, Dummer meant that she learned that solutions to social problems required much more than money, demanding research, study, and comprehensive efforts by a constellation of professionals. This shift in her perspective reflected the dynamic growth of the social sciences at the University of Chicago in this period, and the integral part that settlement house workers and social reformers played in shaping the agenda of these academic disciplines.[10]

In 1908, this connection between social reform and the social sciences was cemented when Dummer became a founder and trustee of the Chicago School of Civics and Philanthropy. This school played a monumental role in shaping the generation of women social scientists who would go on to formulate public policy, reform legislation, and staff-growing governmental bureaucracies. According to one historian, at the Chicago School "female reformers inscribed their progressive commitments on the profession of social work, and . . . were then able to socialize aspiring, younger women into the culture of reform."[11] The Chicago School represented a great push forward in the advancement of the field of social work, and Dummer's help with its founding was just the beginning of her significant contributions to the field and the female reform agenda that shaped it in this period.

After making financial contributions to the NCLC and establishing herself as a sympathetic philanthropist within the reform community in Chicago, Dummer was asked to serve on the board of the Illinois JPA. Through her work in the JPA she became involved with (and critical of) the juvenile court and the entire juvenile justice system. In 1899, Cook County (Chicago) established the first juvenile court in the country. Juvenile courts then spread to many other cities throughout the country, and were considered "one of the most significant of Progressive penal reforms."[12] The courts had admirable aims: to remove youths from the adult criminal justice system, to use social scientific methods to assess the causes of "delinquent" behavior, and to focus on rehabilitation rather than punishment. Dummer's involvement with the courts reflects the high hopes of its creators; she had abiding faith in the contribution that social science and the state would make to understanding and mitigating the causes of delinquency.

Despite the innovations of the juvenile court, from Dummer's perspective, the treatment of delinquent young people was still based primarily on a repressive and punitive model rather than a rehabilitative one. Dummer fiercely objected to the mark imposed on delinquents, whose categorization as "feeble-minded" or "subnormal" was rarely based on adequate scientific research. She dedicated a great deal of money, energy, and thought to undermining hereditarian explanations for behavior. In 1909, with this goal in mind, she helped to create and provided funding for the Juvenile Psychopathic Institute at the Juvenile Court of Chicago. This institute, headed by psychiatrist William Healy, collected data on the delinquents that came through the court system, and was the first of its kind in the United States.[13]

Dummer was especially concerned about the girls who entered the juvenile justice system, who she believed faced particularly difficult obstacles. Many historians have pointed out that humanitarian aims were often undermined by the courts' increased and sometimes inappropriate regulation of the behavior of largely female working-class girls and young women. Mary Odem has shown that, while professional women succeeded in creating a "maternal justice system," that system "continued to subject young women and girls to arrest and to stringent methods of control for sexual misbehavior."[14] Female delinquents almost always made their way to the juvenile court because of sexual misconduct, and many were pregnant as they passed through its halls.[15] Girls who were raped, turned out of their homes, promised marriage, and then left with illegitimate children, or who worked as prostitutes, filled the courtroom.

Dummer's exposure to these vulnerable and exploited girls significantly shaped her interpretation of the politics of maternal welfare. Specifically, while most reformers in her circle saw marriage as the solution to the illegitimacy problem, she rejected the common procedure of forcing marriage on pregnant young women.[16] In holding this position, Dummer found herself at odds with most of her contemporaries. She wrote, "This insisting upon a continued mating of two young persons, who, without love, would bring into the world more unhappy children, made a mockery of marriage. Seeking a solution of these tragedies led into a miry road, but one found pioneers making it possible."[17]

Dummer's frustration with the juvenile justice system in Chicago—one of the most advanced in the country—led her to search for a way to secure protection and justice for the unmarried mother and her child. In 1913 she sailed to Europe for the specific purpose of studying laws concerning women and children. Dummer's interest in laws and culture contrasted sharply with Putnam's foci in this same period—clean milk and better prenatal care. This contrast underscores the variety of ways in which reproductive reformers interpreted women's most pressing needs. Their prewar orientations and choices would carry through and provide clues to the trajectories of their political paths: Putnam moved toward an increasingly medical assessment of the needs of mothers and babies, while Dummer moved from an interest in radical social policy as a means of guarding against maternal victimization toward psychological theories that explained and attempted to treat individual mothers. Significantly, both directions ultimately would make relations with the CB problematic.

A forward written by Havelock Ellis for a book by Swedish feminist Ellen Key first alerted Dummer to Dr. Helene Stöcker and her German radical sex reform group, the *Bund für Mutterschutz und Sexualreform* (Federation for the Protection of Motherhood and Sexual Reform, or BfM).[18] Dummer made a trip to Berlin to meet with Stöcker and to learn more about her innovative ideas surrounding motherhood, sexuality, and marriage. Stöcker was one of the first in a long line of radical thinkers to whom Dummer turned for fresh ideas and inspiration. By the end of her life, Dummer had collected, compiled, and sifted through information from some of the finest and most progressive minds of her era.

Established in 1904, Stöcker's BfM sought to protect and improve the lives of unwed mothers and illegitimate children and to reform sexuality. Stöcker developed an ideological agenda for the BfM that attempted to connect the goals of feminism with an exaltation of motherhood and an explicit critique of traditional marital relations. Her vision consisted of a "New Morality" that sought simultaneously to revolutionize and sanctify motherhood. Stöcker wanted motherhood to be a source of fulfillment and respect for women. Her stress on transforming sexual ethics was framed by a critique of conventional morality that endorsed motherhood only for married women.[19]

On a more practical level, the BfM involved itself with the creation and administration of remarkably comprehensive sex counseling centers where women could get advice on child rearing, contraception, childbirth, breast-feeding, and prenatal care. Atina Grossmann's description of the services available at these centers underscores the truly holistic character of reproductive reform that existed in Weimar Germany:

Explicitly conceived as centers for the protection of women, the clinics also provided aid in cases of wife battering, child abuse, drug addiction, alcoholism, incest, rape, suicide, disturbed children, infertility, overcrowded housing, evictions, and unemployment; in addition they made referrals for therapeutic abortions and sterilizations. Services included home visits and family counselling, childbirth and infant-care classes, complete medical exams, laboratory tests, dental care, education in hygiene, nutrition and physical fitness, even advice on comfortable clothing and home furnishings—in short, everything to decrease infant mortality, illegitimacy, and illegal abortion and to ensure healthy offspring in a healthy family.[20]

Dummer recalls in her autobiography that Stöcker was unknown to any social workers in Chicago, and that those in Berlin, "assured me it would not be worth while to meet with her."[21] As was typical of Dummer, she rejected these secondhand opinions and sought an interview with the philosopher who would forever alter, crystallize, and radicalize her position on the unwed mother and illegitimate child. Years later, she described Stöcker in her autobiography as the "philosopher who had delved deep below the surface of things [and] opened to me the way by which women might climb to a future which would refuse to permit the wastage of women's lives found today."[22]

Through Dummer's introduction to the eclectic politics of the BfM, she was able to imagine a reproductive reform agenda that incorporated both a "health" and a "rights" orientation and that sought to protect all mothers. In 1916, Dummer wrote an essay on feminism in which she expressed her *Mutterschutz* ideas. Highlighting her distance from the Victorian moral code, she rejected the notion that "a woman's life may be ruined because of one mistake." In this piece she also attempted to make the plight of the unwed mother a part of the feminist agenda, arguing that the predicaments of all women were inextricably bound together. She cogently wove the issues of prostitution and illegitimacy together when she wrote, "if the unmarried mothers were given comfort and courage instead of condemnation, the ranks of prostitutes would be depleted."[23] Here Dummer's distinctive analysis begins to take shape as she highlights the plight of the most vulnerable, and links issues of maternity and sexuality with economic and cultural concerns.

Dummer's philosophy, based on the sexual politics of the BfM, echoed concurrent calls for "free love" in the United States. Despite Dummer's thoroughly "respectable" status as a wealthy philanthropist, her views had much in common with contemporary anarchist and socialist rhetoric. Criticism of the institution of marriage and innovative sexual reform politics had become an important part of the socialist agenda by the 1910s.[24] Mari Jo Buhle has argued that the new generation of Socialists in the early twentieth century looked more toward sexologist Edward Carpenter than to Karl Marx to find the "true basis of Socialism."[25] For example, in Emma Goldmann's *Mother Earth* one could find articles that insisted that a child could not be legitimized through marriage, but, rather, that "its birth and presence are the only legitimization that can be bestowed." Despite the commitment of many U.S. socialists and radicals to women's liberation in this period, Dummer never identified herself with either group.[26] She would have found a sympathetic audience for her ideas regarding illegitimacy, marriage, and motherhood amidst radical intellectuals who also looked toward Europe for inspiration. But she perceived herself as a feminist and as part of the mainstream reform community, and never flirted with Marxism.[27]

From Berlin, Stöcker pointed Dummer to Norway, where an innovative piece of legislation dealing with the rights of illegitimate children was being introduced in the Parliament by Johan Castberg, Minister of the Department of Commerce and Social Affairs. Years later, Julia Lathrop would describe this piece of legislation, passed in 1915, "as the first complete national recognition of the inherent right of the child to nurture, protection, and education, irrespective of his parentage."[28] In Norway, Dummer succeeded in complementing her theoretical discoveries with a legal model for protecting mothers and children.

Castberg's law was the most progressive piece of legislation regarding the status of illegitimate children and unwed mothers in the Western world. The law gave illegitimate children equal rights under the law, equal rights to their father's name, and equal rights to inheritance. More specifically, the law stated that fathers should give equal support to illegitimate and legitimate children, that mothers were entitled to financial compensation for loss of earning capacity due to pregnancy and child care, and proper public authorities would collect the money.

The Norwegian law was innovative in two principle ways. First, it sought to eliminate the legal distinction between legitimate and illegitimate children. Second, it gave the state more responsibility and authority over illegitimacy proceedings. This latter facet of the law spelled out a radically increased role for the state to play in the heretofore private family drama of illegitimacy. The Norwegian state was taking on a new responsibility on behalf of unwed mothers and illegitimate children to sue for paternity, and to determine and collect support. Previously, only the mother of the child in question could bring forward a paternity suit, and social stigma often hampered this process. In the United States, the legal system itself discouraged paternity suits by subjecting the mother to criminal charges of lewdness or fornication if she sought paternal support.[29]

In Germany, Dummer had found her theoretical inspiration in Stöcker's BfM, and in Norway she found the exemplary legislation through which to translate her ideas into social change. The legislation combined typical progressive ideas with very atypical ones: on the one hand offering state assistance and protection to vulnerable citizens, and on the other attempting to abolish the stigma associated with illegitimacy (or even the category itself). Upon her return to the United States, Dummer began a campaign to translate and disseminate information on the Norwegian law in order to educate the U.S. public, and, especially, the female reform community in Chicago, on the latest trends in illegitimacy legislation. In order to accomplish her goals, she sought the help of U.S. author and feminist activist Katharine Anthony (1877–1965).

In 1915, Anthony published *Feminism in Germany and Scandinavia*, in which she strove to introduce her American audience to the innovations of continental feminists in the arena of social, sexual, and economic reform. Dummer read this work with excitement, as she recognized that she and Anthony had "discovered" and been converted to the very same ideas and people abroad. The similarity of the women's focus and agenda was uncanny. Both women not only shared a belief in the need for legislative reform along the lines of the Norwegian law, but found their feminism thoroughly shaped by their contact with the BfM.[30] Upon reading *Feminism in Germany and Scandinavia*, Dummer wrote to Anthony's publisher for her address. Her initial letter of introduction began a twenty-year relationship during which Dummer became Anthony's close friend and patron.[31]

In *Feminism in Germany and Scandinavia*, Anthony pointed to the Anglo-American tendency in feminism to define equality in purely political terms, offering the Germans and Scandinavians as an alternative model. The continental feminists, rather than focusing on enfranchisement, emphasized the need to reform social values in order to appreciate the contribution that women made to society through motherhood. Anthony wrote, "In short the struggle for political liberty has fallen to the share of the English and American women and the fight for moral autonomy has fallen to the share of the German and Scandinavian women."[32]

Anthony argued that, while the question of illegitimacy had scarcely been broached in the United States, it was one of the most widely discussed problems in foreign countries, especially with the onset of World War I. Anthony was especially impressed with BfM and argued for the logic of its position regarding sexuality, marriage, and motherhood: "The beginning of the twentieth century brought forth an organized movement which encouraged skepticism toward the Lutheran sex code and championed the victims of this code, the unmarried mothers and the illegitimate child. The *Mutterschutz* idea was the natural historical corrective of an exclusively theological and proprietary marriage."[33]

According to Anthony, the illegitimate child faced three major disadvantages: social stigma, economic hardship, and anonymous paternity. The last two disadvantages could be tackled through constructive legislation, and indeed this political work was being accomplished in Norway through Castberg's law. The social stigma would be dispelled through the spread of the new morality espoused by sex reform groups like the BfM.

In Dummer's first letter to Anthony she wrote that she had "considered organizing an American branch of the *Bund für Mutterschutz*," in order to coax American feminists in the direction of their German and Scandinavian counterparts.[34] Dummer decided that an education and propaganda campaign would be the most logical first step in creating a climate favorable to Castberg-type legislation in the United States. Her faith in education and the power of enlightened public opinion was one of the hallmarks of Progressive-Era reform. Dummer was optimistic that Castberg-type legislation would garner support in the United States from "social workers, probation officers and all interested in Juvenile Court," and she believed that "a strong body of public opinion favorable to it could be easily developed."[35] Anthony was just as optimistic, writing, "I believe thoroughly that the work of the BfM could be duplicated in this country."[36] Neither woman could have predicted the resistance these ideas would face in the United States.

In 1916, Dummer invited Anthony to Chicago to give lectures on the subject of her book before various women's clubs. After Anthony's lectures in Chicago, and the dissemination of 500 copies of the translated Castberg law, Dummer was contacted by four local women's clubs who asked for her help in introducing a similar bill in the Illinois legislature. However, Dummer limited herself to propaganda and education as a matter of personal preference. "I shall leave legislation in the matter to those willing to tie red tape," she said. "My energy must go into securing a more enlightened public opinion."[37] Here, Dummer's penchant for addressing "the big picture" begins to emerge clearly. Fascinated by new ideas and hopeful for social transformation, she shied away from the official sphere of politics, where timidity and formalities seemed to prevail. Dummer's disposition regarding legislation and bureaucracy would be among the important factors that kept her out of positions of power. It was a difficult position for her to maintain over the next few years, as important social changes seemed to be predicated on dealing with both legislation and red tape.

Dummer and Anthony soon learned that, despite the support of a few local women's groups, their commitment to the unwed mother and illegitimate child remained at odds with mainstream progressive reformers. The U.S. response to rising European illegitimacy rates was not monolithic, but very few women reformers were sympathetic to *Mutterschutz* ideas. For example, feminist theorist Charlotte Perkins Gilman was openly critical of, "[T]hose few extreme radicals among Feminists who have been most valiantly upholding the 'right to motherhood.' The position of these ladies . . . is that an unmarried woman has "the right" to bear a child if she so chooses. No consideration of the father's right to share in his child's care, support, education, and society is offered; nor of the child's right to a father, to a family, to a normal position in the world. Only the woman's right to be a mother, at her own good pleasure, is advanced."[38] Gilman derided "the extreme radicals" for their naïve romanticization of motherhood, along with their excessive interest in sex, and offered instead a vision of womanhood that was more "human" than "female."[39]

Mainstream progressive reform efforts to deal with illegitimacy consisted largely of efforts to "elevate" mothers into the "respectable class" through marriage. For example, Dr. Lucy Waite of the *Liberal Review*, along with other reformers and settlement house workers, framed a bill that would have forced marriage after the birth of a child. In an effort to convert Dummer to this position, Waite wrote, "The more I study the subject, and the more bills they try to get up on the subject of illegitimacy avoiding the marriage principle the more I am convinced that the 'parentage-marriage' bill is the only logical solution of the subject. To my mind the child is the only excuse for having marriage laws at all. What interest would the State have in the personal relations of men and woman if it were not for the child?"[40] Waite believed that state responsibility for children translated into a need for state-sanctioned and recognized relations between parents. This type of legislation would ostensibly give the government the opportunity to intercede on the child's behalf and eliminate the entire problem of illegitimacy by making all children legitimate through the subsequent marriage of their parents. However, it still left the child of unwed parents unrecognized and unreachable by the state. It also failed to pose a real challenge to the institution of marriage. According to Dummer, such a law would make a mockery of marriage and, more significantly, perpetuate the distinction between women of the "respectable" class—that is, mothers who were married—and unmarried mothers.

In a letter to Paul Kellogg's *Survey* magazine, Dummer explained the problems with Waite's position, saying, "Recently a bill was suggested by which, at the birth of a child, the father and mother became automatically man and wife. The framers of the bill acknowledged it did not cover cases of the man already married, and also agreed that in many cases it would be well to proceed at once to secure a divorce, but so held by tradition were their minds that two legal fictions were superior to a simple fact."[41] Thus, Dummer expressed criticism of the elaborate maneuvers being touted as necessary to uphold the social viability of an institution that she believed to be quite flawed.

Dummer found herself at odds with many of the other female reformers who were willing to take on the issue of illegitimacy. Her perspective failed to reflect more conventional moral judgments and idealization of the marital state for women and children. Moved by the misery she had seen in the juvenile court and inspired by the feminism of the BfM, Dummer's rather typical maternalist concern for the welfare of girls, young mothers, and their children was complicated by two decidedly atypical convictions: first, all women's problems stemmed from their victimization under a sexual double standard, and, second, those most harmed by this standard—unwed mothers, prostitutes, and the delinquent girls that would most likely make up the ranks of the former two categories—should be treated with empathy and feminist vigilance. Like Putnam, she harbored certain goals that fit squarely within the mainstream of reproductive health reform. Thus, both women were drawn to the work of the early CB. But both displayed an unconventional orientation that would complicate their relations with the Bureau.

The Children's Bureau first came to the problem of illegitimacy through its efforts at birth registration and studies of infant mortality. Through its first study of the issue in Boston, the CB defined illegitimacy as a problem of child welfare. The CB pointed both to the higher mortality rates among children born out of wedlock and to the tendency for health and welfare problems to be more prevalent among this population, noting that "three-fifths of the illegitimate children born in 1914 reached some local agency in the first year of life."[42] Although this also worried Dummer, she was most concerned with securing a modicum of social justice for these children and their mothers.

The development of the Children's Bureau's policies regarding illegitimacy reflected its reluctance to challenge familial and sexual norms. While Linda Gordon has called the CB campaign for reform of illegitimacy laws "principled and feminist: a campaign against the victimization of women and children by a double standard of sexual morality," Dummer's career suggests a different conclusion.[43] The CB approached the problem of illegitimacy much differently than did Dummer: the former was concerned for the welfare of illegitimate children, whereas the latter was committed to securing justice for the unwed mother. Dummer's feminism encouraged her woman-centered vision; the CB's maternalism was decidedly child-centered.

In the summer of 1916, Dummer lent her translated copy of the Castberg law to Julia Lathrop. Dummer felt confident that she and Lathrop held compatible views regarding the significance of this law. Dummer was excited about the Bureau chief's interest and believed that the CB could play a vital role in shaping both public opinion and public policy in this area. Dummer told Lathrop that she regarded Castberg's law as "the highest ethical thought in the matter" of illegitimacy.[44] Castberg had done more than create a just law; she had illuminated the issue for Dummer and was "eager to have it published and share with others the satisfaction which was mine when Herr Castberg made the matter clear to me."[45]

However, as optimistic as Dummer was about using the power of the CB to get the word out on the Norwegian law, she was conscious of the fact that Lathrop's position as Bureau chief might be a liability. Later in the summer, she wrote to Lathrop about the Castberg law, suggesting "Don't you want to write a paper on the subject for the *Journal of Sociology*—or is it too radical a stand for the head of your Bureau to take?"[46] A few months later, Dummer wrote to Anthony that she had received a "noncommittal statement" from the CB indicating "that they would consider having a translation made" of the Castberg law.[47] Impatient with the timidity of the Bureau, Dummer suggested that Anthony try to publish a piece in the *New Republic* in which she could argue that, "The child welfare workers in this country would be interested in the details of the Norwegian Law and that a translation by the Children's Bureau would be a public service."[48]

Lathrop did not personally oversee or set the agenda for the Bureau's work in the area of illegitimacy. Emma Lundberg, Director of the Children's Bureau's Social Service Division, had a more direct role to play in the Bureau's policy development. If Dummer had been dismayed at Lathrop's noncommittal stance due to her highly visible government position, she was even more concerned about Lundberg's initial disinterest and then her emerging policy agenda. Dummer wrote to Anthony: "It was my impression from the tone of the letter received from Miss Lundberg that they needed some more encouragement to go on with the enterprise."[49]

Emma Lundberg immediately set the tone for the Bureau's involvement in the illegitimacy question by employing Dr. Ernst Freund, professor of jurisprudence and public law at the University of Chicago, to write up a study for the Bureau.[50] As the profession of social work attempted to legitimate itself and its claim to the problem of illegitimacy, great pains were taken to slough off the "do-gooder" image of work in this area, as Regina Kunzel and others have shown.[51] Freund was just the kind of expert that the Bureau thought it needed for its intended analysis of illegitimacy laws. Lundberg's memo to Lathrop in 1916 makes clear this predilection towards dispassionate professionalism, stating that Freund's analysis would be "unquestionably an authoritative piece of work, of much greater value than anything our force could turn out."[52]

While the Bureau considered Freund a valued ally in its struggle for child welfare, Dummer complained to Lathrop that he considered her "point of view one which only may be realized in the far future."[53] Dummer helped and coaxed Freund while he was writing this piece for the Bureau. Upon receiving a letter from him that asked her to explain—indeed, almost defend—her support of Castberg, she wrote, "As the mental process which resulted in my acceptance of the Castberg law covered a period of eight years of study and pondering and discussion, I can hardly give it in a letter . . . If you have not seen Miss Anthony's book on feminism in Scandinavia and Germany, I should be glad to lend it to you. Her review of the *Mutterschutz* movement leads to an appreciation of the Norwegian legislation."[54] She wrote Anthony about her concerns, saying, "Professor Freund has a fine mind and is a charming man, but so far as women are concerned he does not understand whither we are tending. I am impressed with the need of bringing before a wider public your vision."[55] Here Dummer begins to distinguish her perspective from the one developed by Freund and accepted by the CB. Her concern was that, although Freund would consider the welfare of children in his examination of legislative trends, he would not recognize how closely illegitimacy laws were bound with women's rights and status. One historian has argued that, for the Children's Bureau, "the rights and protection of the unwed mother devolved from those of her child."[56] For Dummer, on the other hand, a woman's right to motherhood and recognized status as a mother compelled the state to help her. Dummer did not begin with the child as the starting point and build a political reform agenda around it. Indeed, she and Anthony found themselves at odds with the majority of illegitimacy reformers who used "motherhood and children's needs as the major legitimate metaphor with which to discuss women's interests in the political realm."[57]

❧❦

While Dummer grew frustrated with the CB's emerging position on illegitimacy reform, she maintained an alliance with the Bureau and its chief,

Julia Lathrop, through her work with a wartime agency that aimed to stop prostitution and the spread of sexually transmitted diseases among servicemen. Like many progressive reformers, Dummer viewed the war as an unfortunate occurrence that might nevertheless provide opportunities to advance new ideas for social progress. Mothers' pensions and illegitimacy were now part of public discourse in the United States, and the government began taking a more active role in these and related "private" family issues. Two months after President Woodrow Wilson declared war on Germany, Dummer asked Anthony in a letter, "Are you oppressed by the war or can you see emerging out of its horror a new world?"[58] Dummer hoped that the crisis of the war would call attention to questions of state responsibility and social welfare. She wrote, "Although Red Cross and Defense matters may for a time side track interest in home matters, . . . more and more does the European situation show us that the whole problem of motherhood and the relation of the child to the state needs scientific consideration."[59] Dummer became part of that scientific consideration through her involvement with the Commission on Training Camp Activities (CTCA). Although briefly distracting her from her efforts at illegitimacy reform, this work was a logical outgrowth of her prewar work in the arena of juvenile justice and, specifically, female delinquency.

In April 1917, Raymond B. Fosdick was appointed chairman of the CTCA.[60] The Commission was created to reduce the incidence of sexually transmitted disease among U.S. servicemen. The guiding philosophy of the CTCA was that women were the harbingers of disease and impurity and were consequently sapping the strength of the U.S. armed forces. The CTCA's procedures displayed a blatant double standard in that they called for the arrest or incarceration of women for spreading venereal disease, while offering soldiers medical treatment. According to historian Allen Brandt, "the massive arrests and detention of prostitutes raised a basic conundrum of public health: How far could a government go in the name of science and hygiene to abridge the rights of those who might threaten the greater good?"[61] Specifically, Brandt refers to the tendency of the U.S. government to view the war effort and the health of the armed forces as "the greater good" and prostitutes and other women who had sexual relations with soldiers as "the threat."

In September 1917, Fosdick created the Committee on Protective Work for Girls (CPWG). Ostensibly, the CPWG's responsibility was to prevent "delinquency" by keeping women either completely away from training camps, or by aiding them in finding productive, nonthreatening work to do in the vicinity of the camps. He appointed Maude E. Miner of the New York Probation and Protective Association to supervise the activities of this committee. Miner was a pioneer in the movement to create detention homes for female offenders as an alternative to traditional prisons. Julia Lathrop and Ethel Dummer also served on this committee. Here, they forged an alliance against the repressive and sexist policies of the committee, and found common ground in their concern for the war's impact on infants and mothers.

Brandt has argued that the philosophy of the CTCA was not necessarily fed by conservative, military sources, but actually by "Progressive fears of the decline of the family."[62] Similarly, Mary Odem's study of women reformers has led her to argue that, despite honorable intentions, progressive women social workers ultimately "lent their services to the repressive campaign" of incarceration and compulsory examination of suspected venereal disease carriers.[63] Dummer, however, was no typical progressive reformer. Her time in Europe had exposed her to radical sexual reform politics to which few U.S. feminists and reformers had been exposed, let alone converted. Dummer did not believe that women were the source of familial decline or the source of the health problems of the U.S. Armed Forces. She was not horrified by children born out of wedlock, disgusted by prostitutes, or convinced that women who engaged in sex outside marriage were feebleminded or fallen. While the CPWG dedicated itself to reducing sexually transmitted disease, illicit sexual activity, and illegitimacy, Dummer sought to utilize the Committee to promote the rights of delinquent girls, prostitutes, and unmarried mothers. Her feminism, spiced with a sexual critique of the social order, made her a maverick among the military and medical men who ran the CTCA, and a progressive voice among the women in the CPWG.

Dummer anticipated some of the prejudices and problems she would face as a member of the CPWG. Granted, when Fosdick asked Dummer to serve on the committee, Dummer wrote back one week later accepting his offer rather graciously. However, she had written another version of this acceptance letter that she ultimately decided not to send to Fosdick. The unsent letter illustrated the internal trepidation with which she embarked on this new project: "Though the work you offer is somewhat appalling in its extent, it is of great interest, and, feeling sure that under Maude Miner it will be not merely repressive, but constructive in a large way, I will serve on the committee."[64] This bolder version of Dummer's acceptance letter illustrates her concern that under the wrong direction the CPWG might exhibit the same problems that plagued the juvenile court system, where punishment often took precedence over efforts to provide compassionate and rehabilitative care.

Dummer, though, had her reasons for accepting the position. Her desire to learn more about the women and girls who had fascinated her since her involvement with the JPA proved very strong. She decided to join the committee in an effort to gather as much information on the female delinquent, prostitute, and unwed mother as possible. A true believer in the power of scientific investigation, Dummer could not resist the opportunity to collect data on female sexual misconduct. In a letter to Anthony, she expressed both her optimism and her long-term goals: "Though any sort of policing and espionage is distasteful, the amount of good being done through securing medical care, rehabilitation, and education is amazing, and the statistics being gathered will be of untold value."[65]

At this point in her life, Dummer was a believer in bureaucratic efficiency, provided that the policies emanating from the bureaucracy were enlightened. Echoing the sentiments of Elizabeth Putnam in her support of a centralized bureaucracy to coordinate milk inspection, Dummer told Lathrop that she preferred the orders from the War Department in Washington, D.C., "to the hodge podge of the decisions of old-fashioned judges."[66] Thus, envisioning the CPWG as presenting an important social-scientific opportunity, as well as an opportunity to create a humane, centralized policy, Dummer began her brief experiment as a bureaucrat.

In the early days of the CPWG, Dummer and the others tried to advance their own goals along with, or even in spite of, orders from Washington. For example, Julia Lathrop and Dummer attempted to promote maternal health care and the building of reformatories and detention homes that worked toward rehabilitation rather than punishment. These two women cemented their relationship within the CPWG while forging their ambitious "extra-curricular" plans for the postwar period.

During the war, Lathrop was first able to develop and run a visiting nurse program in rural areas, which became the model on which the Bureau later based the organization and administration of Sheppard-Towner. However, funds were not readily available for this particular type of war work, so Lathrop turned to Dummer for financial backing. Dummer responded to her request with enthusiasm, writing, "Your campaign for the care of mothers appeals to me much more than helping to police outskirts of the war training camps, which is, as yet, the only service asked of me."[67] Dummer paid the first year's salary of a visiting nurse in Wyoming, assuring Lathrop that she would "not let anyone else have the satisfaction of helping to carry out this very splendid plan of yours."[68] Thus, Dummer's philanthropy provided the seeds for Sheppard-Towner, following the trajectory of women's political activism from voluntarism and philanthropy to state-sponsored social programs.

By 1918, Fosdick renamed the CPWG the Section on Women and Girls, and put it under the jurisdiction of the Law Enforcement Department of the CTCA. Dummer was alarmed at this change, interpreting it as a clear indication that even more emphasis would now be put on protecting the health of the soldiers rather than the girls and women around the camps. She wrote to Lathrop, "repression and mere law enforcement, especially if it means a return to medical supervision of prostitutes, falls far short of what I had hoped the work of the committee might be."[69] She lamented that the army was willing to spend money on law enforcement, but not on clinics to treat and rehabilitate women.

Among the practices of the CTCA that most enraged Dummer were its encouragement of "war-time marriages," and its attempt to give immunity to servicemen facing paternity suits.[70] These practices not only contradicted one another, but also went against Dummer's sense of justice and morality. They were anathema to all that Dummer stood for at the juvenile court and further cemented her conviction that forced marriages made a mockery of the institution and ruined more lives than they purported to save.

Dummer was not the only member of the CPWG who felt frustrated by Washington's policies regarding the treatment of women. In April 1918, Maude Miner resigned as director of the CPWG. Miner blamed the CTCA for being uninterested in protecting girls, but only in protecting soldiers. Despite Dummer's similar frustration over the work in the CPWG, she would not give up. Her optimism stemmed partially from her belief in the committee's ability to shape public policy during and after the war. In a letter to Binford, Dummer characteristically expressed both her outrage at current policies and her hopes for the future, writing, "Do you not think our Committee should come to some standard of requirement which we may put before the country as a present minimum to be asked for the position of women? Why should women be imprisoned for a disease when a man, as responsible, goes scott free? Why should women be held in the bondage of prostitution because city councils and boards of health are bound up with vice rings? If the world is striving for freedom, is it not time to demand for women not alone political but social rights?"[71] These sentiments typified Dummer's politics, as she consistently tied the plight of the prostitute to that of all women and tried to shift attention toward the social rights of women. Dummer's notion of social rights was both abstract, in that it obliterated the sexual double standard, and practical, in that it obliterated compulsory medical examinations for prostitutes. To work toward both goals, Dummer remained with the wartime commission.

Dummer's decision to remain involved with the CPWG stemmed not just from sentiment and high hopes, but from her commitment to gathering scientific data on the female delinquent. Despite the government's mistreatment of women at that time, she remained confident that information gathered on the female delinquent during the war would inspire an altogether new system of justice when properly analyzed. She envisioned, "a development for our Committee far beyond what our finances permit, and the securing of psychological and sociological data which should be a distinct contribution to the feminist movement."[72]

Perhaps one reason for Dummer's optimism and resiliency in the face of the "military and medical mind" stemmed from her distance from the center of the fray in Washington, D.C. Her official capacity on the committee lasted only a matter of months at which time a tubercular attack led her to rest in California, where she received weekly and monthly reports from field workers.[73] Dummer maintained an involvement with the work of the committee through correspondence. Her fascination with the female delinquent was satisfied by the constant flow of case studies to her home in California throughout the remainder of the war. She poured over these case histories in an effort to find a common link or a clue that would unveil the mystery of the delinquent girl. This data would ultimately aid Dummer in formulating an innovative theory on female delinquency.

After the war, the government dismantled its elaborate public health system. Even as the CPWG lost all of its funding for research and rehabilitation, Dummer refused to give up hope for securing justice for the prostitute and unwed mother. Characteristically optimistic, she wrote to Jessi Binford that, "The withdrawal of the government's financial support will arouse the states and private associations to the establishment of the free clinics with social service which offers personal and friendly encouragement. . . . Although the appropriation was defeated from motives opposed to our work, the action may give the needed stimulus to wiser carrying out of our idea."[74] In addition to placing her hopes in the state legislatures and private organizations, Dummer also believed that women's clubs would take up the banner of the rights for prostitutes and would be crucial in changing public opinion.[75] Dummer and her progressive colleagues could predict neither the rising tide of political conservatism in the postwar period nor the changes in the women's movement after suffrage. Like Elizabeth Putnam, Dummer grew increasingly disillusioned with government bureaucracy and the policies emanating from it in the 1920s. Both women began to view public policies related to women and mothers as misguided in various ways and to various degrees. However, much of Dummer's frustration stemmed from the government's waning commitment to social welfare and public health, especially for the vulnerable and disadvantaged groups she championed. For Dummer, like most progressives, only the Sheppard-Towner Act stood out in the postwar years as a symbol of prewar hopes for federally funded social welfare services. The end of the war brought disappointment not only with governmental retrenchment in the arena of social welfare, but also with the postwar agenda of the CB. Dummer's feminism is most acutely contrasted with the Bureau's maternalism in the ensuing debate over the nature of illegitimacy reform, a contrast that helps explain her retreat from social policy in the 1920s and 1930s.

☙❦☙

Lathrop conducted a few small, unpublicized meetings in 1917 and 1918 to discuss the effects of the war on children born out of wedlock and to develop a more long-term policy agenda. Dummer was one of twenty people from across the nation that Lathrop invited to Washington, D.C., for the first informal discussion. The Castberg law was one of the pieces of legislation under consideration at these forums.

By 1919 the Children's Bureau was ready to hold larger public conferences to discuss legislation for the protection of children born out of wedlock. The Bureau publicized these forums, which encouraged discussion among social workers, court workers, and lawyers. Two regional conferences on illegitimacy were held in New York and Chicago. The CB's goal was to forge agreement on principles for legislative standards out of which it would draft a model law as a guide for states.

Dummer could not attend these conferences and, according to one friend, was sorely missed by the more progressive element there. Jessi Binford, who had served with both Lathrop and Dummer on the CPWG, wrote that she "would (have) give(n) anything in the world if you could have been here for I feel you would make a contribution that no one else can."[76] As it turned out, the model law was reflective of Dummer's absence.

The law designed by those at the Children's Bureau conferences was finished by 1922 and sent on to the National Conference of Commissioners on Uniform State Laws to create a final version that would be recommended to state legislatures. The uniform law did include some of the most important aspects of the Castberg law: it was based on the principle that parents owed maintenance, education and support to their children regardless of their legal status. However, what got left out of the uniform law was equally important and interesting.

Freund reported that during the conferences there were many objections to improving what he called the "status rights" of illegitimate children—

e.g., making children born of null and void marriages legitimate. The objection was that muddying the boundaries between children born in and out of wedlock would "undermin[e] one of the pillars of our social order."[77] Freund went on to explain that the decision to leave out the controversial status question was a pragmatic measure. "[O]n reflection," he said, "the Committee decided to drop . . . the entire article dealing with status rights . . . the sentiment that was revealed was taken as a timely and symptomatic warning. If influential members of the Conference felt so strongly that traditional rules of the marriage law should not be disturbed, the same attitude was sure to appear later on in state legislatures with the possible effect of wrecking the entire measure in a number of states."[78] The uniform law thus abandoned the status issue and became "a support measure pure and simple."[79]

Freund claimed that he was sympathetic to the more radical ideas put forth by Castberg, "under which the father of every illegitimate child is compelled by the state to assume the full obligation that is owing to a lawful child," but argued that these ideas did not seem pragmatic. Louise Bowen, director of the JPA in Chicago, agreed with Freund. Evidently skeptical of the practicality of the status provisions, she asked, "Can legislation, unless it overwhelmingly represents contemporaneous public sentiment, overcome the social sanctions and accepted points of view which it has taken centuries to develop?"[80] Dummer, however, remained quite unsatisfied with these compromises. To her, the status question was central to securing social justice for both unwed mothers and their children. She sought to obliterate the legal distinctions between the legitimate and illegitimate child in an effort to collapse the distinction between respectable and fallen women. Although glad that the legislation spelled out an expanded responsibility for fathers and the state, Dummer lamented that the truly innovative and radical elements of Castberg had been excluded from the uniform law.

The women of the Children's Bureau considered the issue of status, but ended up supporting a policy of improving maintenance rights for children born out of wedlock. This is much more than a semantic difference, as the question of status would have directly challenged the institution of marriage by eliminating the legal difference between illegitimate and legitimate children. Initially intrigued by Castberg and flirting with *Mutterschutz* ideas, the CB seemed to want to view illegitimacy as a cultural as well as an economic issue. For example, Lathrop referred to restoring the mother's standing, eliminating laws remaining on state statute books that revealed "strange archaic remnants of the most brutal attitude toward women."[81] Ultimately, however, in the postwar period, the CB supported a uniform law that secured funds for children but omitted the issue of their status, rights to inheritance, and rights to their fathers' names. Lundberg felt this omission was completely logical and "desirable in order to carry through the more vital points."[82] She clearly saw the maintenance issue as the vital one, and agreed with Freund that chances were not good for a Castberg-type law.

Dummer's position was supported by a small faction of more radical social workers at the illegitimacy conferences who sought to give children born out of wedlock equal rights and to obliterate all distinctions between legitimate and illegitimate children. However, the majority of reformers did not want to go as far as Castberg, and so presented a formidable obstacle. As one historian has argued, "[F]aced with widespread conservatism, . . . reformers often sacrificed the ideal of equal rights for the easier goal of relieving public and private charity of the burden of a large number of dependent children."[83] This approach is precisely the one that Freund and the Children's Bureau pursued; that is, they abandoned the more difficult goal of attaining equality for illegitimate children, instead pursuing the more palatable call to relieve economic dependency through reform of procedures related to the establishment of paternity and the provision of maintenance funds to children.

In 1920 Emma Lundberg and Katharine Lenroot published *Illegitimacy as a Child Welfare Problem.*[84] In this publication, the authors attempt to stake a claim for the illegitimate child as a pressing welfare issue in the United States. Lundberg and Lenroot chart the unfortunate path of the typical illegitimate child from birth to death: first there is lack of a stable home, financial support, and proper maternal care. This situation leads to poor health, dependence on public support, and abnormal character development. The illegitimate child represented a threat to society as a potential delinquent and drain on public funds; therefore, it was in society's best interest to work toward reversing this downward spiral. These dual goals—humanitarian and economic—were articulated by Lenroot and Lundberg in the following passage: "The increasing tendency to exert every effort to conserve child life results from the recognition of the obligation of society to insure for all children a childhood as nearly normal as possible and to develop them into useful and valuable members of the community."[85]

Dummer conceived of illegitimacy as an issue that adversely affected both women and children. Her concerns about women's status and infant and child welfare came together in her campaign to spread information on the Norwegian illegitimacy law and to rethink this issue from a feminist perspective. Dummer's introduction to the radical sex reformers of the

BfM led her to characterize the unwed mother not as a fallen or immoral woman, but, rather, as the victim of a merciless sexual double standard. Dummer offered a different—some would argue more nuanced, others more naïve—reading of what was at stake in reforming illegitimacy laws. For her, the problem was not merely one of coaxing the state to extend its protection and support to this unfortunate population of children. She hoped, instead, for a new way of understanding, respecting, and celebrating motherhood in all its forms. This vision of a new morality was precisely what bureaucrats, most social workers, and crafters of legislation wanted to omit from legislative reform. Thus, the laws that were created sought to keep these children alive and cared for, but never challenged the stigma attached to children born out of wedlock or their mothers.

The development and shape of the Bureau's position regarding illegitimacy raises a number of questions. Some historians have interpreted its policies as a reaction to the conservative political climate.[86] Many historians, including Muncy, Sheila Rothman, and Molly Ladd-Taylor, have shown that the Bureau had to narrow its focus on many controversial issues in order to survive in the first two decades. Clearly, that interpretation captures one aspect of the story. The CB, like Dummer, was initially intrigued by the Castberg law, but eventually backed away from its more radical implications. The right to have a child out of wedlock, like the right to control whether and when to have children through artificial contraception, was not a right the CB was willing to defend in the interwar years. Of course, one could argue that the CB's mandate was to investigate and report on matters related to child, not maternal, welfare. However, the CB's own studies proved that illegitimate children and children born to mothers who were ill, poor, or had too many other children experienced higher rates of morbidity and mortality. These circumstances certainly made the right to birth control and the rights of illegitimate children potentially valid arenas of activity. However, both of these reproductive rights fell outside the CB's purview, for it conceived of itself as a defender of the traditional family in the conservative 1920s. Facing opposition to Sheppard-Towner, accusations of teaching birth control in its maternal health programs, and cries that it was seeking to nationalize child rearing and undermine family life, the CB shielded itself by disassociating from certain causes. The CB was well aware of what it was leaving out when it helped formulate a legislative model for the states to follow in reforming their laws in this area. The staff of the Bureau was conscious of making political choices and compromises.

However, it would be simplistic to argue that the CB's stance on illegitimacy was purely strategic or even unprincipled. It pursued and won the passage of better maintenance laws for children born out of wedlock, which was perfectly in keeping with its ideology of progressive maternalism and sensitivity to the economics of mother-work. Among the most important differences between Dummer and the CB was their perception of why illegitimacy presented a problem: was maintenance, on the one hand, or status, on the other, to blame? Their interpretations of the nature of the problem laid the foundation for the different legislative and policy paths they ultimately chose. If the issue was defined as one of child health, support and education, the emphasis would fall on the economic rights of children, and the legal reforms would center around maintenance laws. If the problem was perceived as issue of status, the goal would be to eliminate the legal distinction between legitimate and illegitimate children. This latter position incorporates a direct critique of the institution of marriage and the sexual double standard. Originally based on European *Mutterschutz* ideas, it asserts that women are providing a service in mothering, that all women deserve state support, and, finally, that women can create families with or without men's help. The former position, focusing on maintenance, articulates none of those social and cultural critiques.

The ideological distance between Dummer and the CB can be also seen in their perspectives on maternal endowments and the family wage. Endowments attracted Dummer because they would serve two functions that were important to her: creating a system of direct state support to women, and undermining the patriarchal family structure. On the other hand, the CB endorsed mothers' pensions as a way to uphold gender conventions; these pensions could simultaneously keep mothers out of the workforce and avoid the sticky issue of childcare provision. As in the case of its stand on illegitimacy reform, the CB focused on getting financial support to needy children in ways that did not challenge prevailing gender and familial roles.[87]

Despite the fact that, by 1919, a total of thirty-nine states had mothers' pensions in varying forms, only Michigan legislation explicitly included unmarried mothers. Even by the 1930s, widows—traditionally perceived as the most deserving recipients of aid—still comprised 82 percent of mothers receiving government aid. According to Mark H. Leff, mothers' pensions were so staunchly supported in part because the program "promised to be cheap and morally uplifting."[88] Women who would receive pensions needed to behave "properly" so as to ensure that the program would not encourage immoral practices. Susan Tiffin has argued that, "The mothers' pension scheme typified the various and often conflicting attitudes of the Progressive movement of child welfare. . . . Reformers envisioned that the welfare of thousands of children and mothers would be guaranteed by the creation of state funds to provide regular relief. At the same time, their anxiety for the stability of American society undermined the adequate application of this relief and made it conditional upon the assumptions of middle-class behavioral norms."[89] For these reasons, legislation in the United States fell far short of Dummer's vision, as it rejected social and ethical transformation and used the promise of government money to reinforce white middle-class American values.

In 1920 Dummer wrote, "While mankind accepts economics as the basis of life, financial recognition only will secure realization of the value of motherhood. . . . *for the self respect of the mother,* economic independence is a necessity as for the welfare of the child."[90] Not surprisingly, the more mainstream discussions of mothers' pensions rarely mentioned maternal self-respect. Once again, Dummer added a feminist twist to what was otherwise considered a child welfare issue. She argued that maternal endowments would not only save and improve the lives of children, but would also replace a patriarchal financial arrangement with a more systematic and just social welfare program.

In the pre- and postwar era, many child welfare reformers fought simultaneously for mothers' pensions and a family wage, as either strategy seemed to promise protection of children in the family. Dummer defied this tendency and specifically argued for maternal endowment as a corrective or countermeasure to a family wage system. She rejected the idea that, by ensuring a family wage for the head of the household, women and children would be adequately cared for. Dummer was part of the group of reformers identified by Wendy Sarvasy, whose, "feminist analysis . . . offered a way to counter the hegemonic familisitic framework that assumed that social programs should strengthen only the father-headed model of the family."[91] Her aim to abolish the distinction between children born in and out of marriage went hand in hand with a commitment to a comprehensive system of maternal endowment. Dummer acknowledged that freeing women and children from social stigma would be meaningless if they were not also guaranteed a minimum standard of living.

While the Children's Bureau supported mothers' pensions, which were means-tested, morals-tested, and ultimately stigmatizing, Dummer envisioned a universal system of support for all mothers. She and Katharine Anthony preferred the European term "maternal endowment" to the watered-down U.S. version, "mothers' pensions." Making a clear distinction between a system of pensions and a system of endowment, Katharine Anthony argued, "that the services of the mother in the home are worth a remuneration from the State," and that "it should not be paid as a pension or bounty."[92] Dummer and Anthony argued that state support actually facilitated women's independence because this support would undermine women's dependence within the patriarchal family. Without a feminist critique of the traditional male breadwinner family, maternal endowments were usually seen as creating dependence, rather than relieving it.

Despite disagreements over both maternal endowments and illegitimacy reform, Dummer maintained a cordial relationship with the women who ran the CB throughout the 1920s. Whereas Putnam saw Sheppard-Towner as a step in the wrong direction, Dummer sent Lathrop a note offering "Hearty congratulations to you upon the Senate action on your bill." She went on to flatter the chief by comparing her to both Mary Wollstonecraft and Olympe de Gouges, arguing that neither woman "has done more for women than you have."[93] Here, Dummer's comments once again reveal her orientation; while Sheppard-Towner was designed and pitched both on Capitol Hill and to the U.S. public as a plan to lower infant mortality and improve the health of America's babies, Dummer interpreted its value in terms of its impact on women's lives.

❦

In the 1920s, discouraged by the CB and the public policy emanating from it, Dummer moved back to her initial interest in the causes and treatment of female delinquency. Unable to compete with the professionals who shaped maternal and infant welfare policies, she concentrated instead on funding particular people and projects that promised to advance her goals. One of her major contributions in this area involved a grant of $10,000 to William I. Thomas for research on delinquency. Even after her experience on the CPWG, Dummer held fast to the faith that social science research would light a path toward humane and effective social policy.[94] The official contract between Dummer and Thomas illustrates the political motives behind her philanthropic gesture: "This study is primarily to gather and interpret such data as shall lead to less unjust and futile treatment than is at present accorded so-called delinquent women, changing not only public opinion, but especially altering procedure in our courts, jails, and hospitals: But it is hoped that it may also tend toward a better understanding of human relations and indicate marriage standards based scientifically on biology and psychology rather than on a past system of economics."[95] Thus, Dummer's retreat from the arena of public policy did not signal a lessening of her comprehensive critique of marriage, nor of her commitment to social justice. The book that evolved from this research, *The Unadjusted Girl* (1923) is considered a classic text of the Chicago School.

Dummer's role in the making of *The Unadjusted Girl* went beyond philanthropy. She provided Thomas with the data she had gathered during the war, and freely shared her unique perspective with him. By this time, Dummer had begun to develop her own theory regarding female delinquency, one that grew out of her personal experience with delinquents and wide reading on the subject. Dummer brought together two basic ideas: first, criminologists considered many prostitutes and sexual delinquents to be feeble-minded, and, second, postwar psychologists were developing various cures and rehabilitative therapies for "shell-shocked" soldiers. Dummer's involvement with delinquent girls had revealed that early sexual experience or abuse was a common factor in many of their lives. Dummer hypothesized that the so-called feeblemindedness or abnormality evident in this population might be due to a sort of "shell shock" or trauma related to their early sexual experience. In other words, Dummer believed that the mental state of delinquent girls and prostitutes was based on circumstantial or social influences, rather than on some innate genetic quality. The implications of this theory were that girls could be cured of "feeblemindedness," and that prostitutes were victims rather than predators who could be reformed. Thomas's work, while not directly incorporating Dummer's theory, certainly emphasized environmental factors in understanding delinquency. Since the publication of his earlier, very influential book *The Polish Peasant in Europe and America* (1918), Thomas had developed a reputation for looking into the varied and complex circumstances that surrounded and shaped personal behavior.[96]

Both Dummer's and Thomas's orientation toward the cultural norms and environmental factors that victimized women reflected a shift in the field of social work toward psychotherapy and case work. It is not surprising that Dummer found much inspiration in new psychological theories that emphasized human complexity, resiliency, and the centrality of sexuality to human behavior. Since her days at the Juvenile Court, Dummer had rejected the damaging labels attached to female offenders and sought a more humane system of diagnosis and treatment. Psychoanalytic theory held out promise in both of these arenas. It appealed to her belief in the ability of people to improve themselves, while also providing a strong defense against putative treatment of juvenile offenders. It also provided an overt critique of sexual repression and an implicit critique against the sexual double standard.

Although historians often interpret the trend in social work away from large-scale policy goals and toward case work as a retreat from social reform and a reflection of the growing conservatism of the field, Dummer's attraction to psychology lends itself to a different interpretation. In light of the fact that large-scale social reform seemed increasingly unlikely to be accomplished in the 1920s, progressives searched for alternative ways of supporting and protecting the vulnerable and disadvantaged. In other words, what progressives could no longer accomplish through political activism, they tried to achieve through case work and the therapeutic model.

Penologist Miriam Van Waters, whose career was advanced through Dummer's patronage, provides a model of a social worker who moved in similar directions in the interwar years.[97] By the 1920s, Dummer was spending less time in Chicago and more time in California. While in California, she became associated with an innovative school, nicknamed "El Retiro," for delinquent girls—including unwed mothers—run by Van Waters. Van Waters developed a new type of rehabilitative and educational therapy in her establishment in Los Angeles, California, and was considered the leading figure in female penology in the interwar years. Van Waters became another long-term recipient of Dummer's personalized brand of philanthropy. She gave Dummer credit for turning the seed of an idea into a tangible and permanent project through her foresight, compassion, and wealth.

Van Waters, like Dummer, rejected the notion that female delinquents were inherently bad or untreatable. In words that echoed Dummer's deepest convictions, Van Waters implored, "let us let go of the concept of the moral judgement and seek as patiently as social physicians must, the causes that underlie behavior."[98] As an agent of the Boston Children's Aid Society, she began to recognize the mistreatment of female delinquents and the tendency for girls' crimes to be of a moral or sexual nature. In 1917 Van Waters was appointed superintendent of the Los Angeles County Juvenile Home; in 1919 she took over El Retiro. El Retiro was "founded to relieve the emergencies of World War I when the port of Los Angeles was closed to sailors because of vice conditions."[99] Insofar as it was part of the national effort to "protect" girls, the reformatory attracted Dummer's attention. Van Waters described the establishment as a "preventorium" where self-government, vocational choices, and attention to girls' emotional lives and well-being marked its departure from the norm. In Van Waters Dummer had found another kindred spirit upon whom she bestowed affection and funds. According to her biographer, Van Waters dedicated her life to securing "maternal justice" and saw her role "as a charismatic counselor whose psychological insights could help uplift souls."[100] Dummer helped Van Waters realize this vision by funding her hiring of a staff psychologist to assist in the treatment of the girls at El Retiro.

Two years after funding William I. Thomas's *Delinquent Girl*, she offered Van Waters the chance to study schools for delinquent girls throughout the country. At Dummer's memorial service in 1954, Van Waters recalled the exciting research. "Mrs. Dummer sent me out over the nation. I went to twenty-six states surveying reform schools, making recommendations to the Federal government for the granting of aid to those with constructive policies."[101] Specifically, Van Waters pointed to Dummer's involvement with the federal government during the war as a significant influence on her career. "When we get combined with that compassion, awareness and keenness of what government has set up and what government is doing, confidence in the scientific process, then you have indeed a pioneer in social invention."[102] The result of Van Waters's research was a study entitled "Where Girls Go Right," published in the *Survey Graphic* in 1922. From then on, Van Waters continued to receive support from Dummer and published two books, *Youth in Conflict* (1925) and *Parents on Probation* (1927) with her financial help. These widely read books helped to promote new psychological explanations of female delinquency.[103]

While Dummer's patronage influenced the shape of postwar academic research on and treatment of female delinquency, Dummer enjoyed less success in the arenas of public policy and public opinion. Dummer viewed delinquency and illegitimacy as part of a larger agenda to secure justice for all women, but her perspective would never gain ascendancy among the mainstream female reform community. Her efforts to aid the unwed mother and her child through both financial support and transformation of the moral code never had the impact on public policy that she had hoped for. The progressive maternalists who shared her concern for mothers and children did not share her feminist politics; the feminists in organizations like the National Women's Party who had toyed with the idea of maternal endowment began to abandon motherhood rhetoric for an almost exclusive focus on equal opportunities for women outside the home.[104] After years of struggling for this societal change of heart, Dummer told Anthony, "It often puzzles me that people are astonished when I differentiate between marriage laws and sexual ethics."[105]

By the 1930s Dummer, now in her seventies, was turning increasingly away from big philanthropic projects and toward familial matters. Although several of the women who had served with her during World War I on the CPWG became involved with the creation and administration of New Deal policy, Dummer remained noticeably absent from this select group. Dummer's status was no longer enough to provide her with opportunities in the government, for civil service reform and women's increased educational opportunities in the 1920s meant that only a small group of female professionals would ascend to these much sought-after positions. According to Estelle Freedman, "although she was extremely well informed and articulate, Dummer felt self conscious about her lack of a college education."[106] Without a professional degree but with an impressive fortune and a deep social conscience, Dummer acted in a supporting role to the female dominion in child welfare policy that developed over the first two decades of the twentieth century. Although her personal style of philanthropy allowed her to fund the projects and people closest to her heart, she never achieved the political power or authority among her cohort that her wealth might have promoted. A clear example of this supporting role can be seen in her relationship with the Chicago School. Dummer was a founding trustee of the school, yet she remained at the margins of the female dominion fueled by such institutions. While the administrators and faculty of the Chicago School educated students who "often filled positions that permitted them to mold others and to affect public policy,"[107] Dummer's opportunities to influence public policy diminished during the interwar years. Thus, Dummer's funds ironically created and perpetuated the very type of institution that ultimately made her lay expertise obsolete, with its emphasis on scientific training and professionalism.

Characterizing herself as a mystic and an intellectual, Dummer was never comfortable with bureaucracy or formal politics. She admitted that she did not have the stamina and diplomacy necessary for involvement in the political process. Her brief involvement with federal projects during the war allowed her to investigate and develop her ideas on the subject of female delinquency. Therefore, she remained with the wartime committee despite her disappointment with its philosophy and scope. Ultimately, however, the distance between Dummer's vision and the reality of reproductive reform politics discouraged her from direct engagement with the political process. Unlike Putnam, who found a comfortable home in the conservative wing of the Republican Party in the interwar years, no political party incorporated or even tolerated Dummer's vision.

☙❧

Dummer believed that all women (but especially in their role as mothers) were victimized by an oppressive moral code. Following the logic of feminist theorists such as Ellen Key and Helene Stöcker, she believed that motherhood should be supported unconditionally. Dummer once wrote in regard to motherhood, "It is not the occupation but the world's attitude towards it that needs changing."[108] In her mind, the issues of illegitimacy, delinquency, prostitution, and maternal endowments were inextricably linked. Unwed mothers, who often hailed from the ranks of delinquent girls, were simply the mothers most in need of financial support so they would not turn to a life of prostitution. For Dummer, reproductive reform necessitated a commitment to those women on the fringes of social respectability. Helping the most vulnerable and the most victimized would ameliorate the cultural, legal, and economic circumstances that held women down.

Like many progressives and social feminists, Dummer hoped that the state might have a positive impact of women's lives. She advanced a notion of social welfare that included responsibility without runaway power or control, but was disappointed in more mainstream visions of morality and family life. Like the German feminists who inspired her, Dummer advocated unconditional social and economic support for all mothers. She rejected the traditional view of the nuclear family and marriage, thereby challenging many of the underlying premises upon which early twentieth century maternal, child, and family welfare programs were based. Her critique of the family wage system and punitive treatment of unmarried mothers placed her at odds with the moral and economic principles at the core of the mainstream reproductive health reform community, as represented by the Children's Bureau.

Dummer argued against saving the kind of family that perpetuated women's subordination through economic vulnerability and a sexual double standard. In the struggle for power between the family and the state, Dummer equated the former with male authority and saw the latter as a means of relief for women's secondary status. In contrast, Putnam's concern for the family in general, and maternal welfare in particular, did not rest on a commitment to women's equality or liberation. Putnam simply did not interpret maternal and infant welfare as feminist issues that demanded feminist solutions; that is, she did not perceive problems such as maternal mortality emanating from women's lack of power within the family or in society at large.

Dummer's career as a reproductive reformer provides an alternative lens through which to view and interpret white women's political activism in the early twentieth century. While toying with large-scale political and legislative change in the prewar and immediate postwar years, Dummer ultimately rejected the larger political process in favor of personal development and more narrow efforts on behalf of specific portions of the population. Despite high hopes through the 1910s, she could not find a comfortable home for her feminist politics within the liberal state of the 1920s or the activist state of the 1930s. Nor was she able to find a comfortable or formidable role as part of the female dominion in American reform, whose development and peak coincided directly with Dummer's career. Her faith in the power of education rather than legislation, discomfort with lobbying and bureaucratic channels, and controversial feminist ideology made her increasingly less influential in the interwar years, as professionalism took hold in the fields of politics and social reform.

3

"Has the government the right to forbid knowledge?"

MARY WARE DENNETT, EXPEDIENCY,
JUSTICE, AND BIRTH CONTROL

*A*s Elizabeth Putnam and Ethel Dummer each strove to take the infant and maternal welfare movement in new directions—offering alternative interpretations of mothers' needs and how these needs connected to broader social and political issues—the movement to legalize birth control was not without its debates and controversies. Many of these debates centered around similar fundamental questions: What do mothers most need to safeguard their own and their children's health? Which alliances would benefit the movement and what impact would these alliances have? How far could/should the movement go in challenging cultural norms related to family life and, in particular, women's role? Like the reproductive health movement, the reproductive rights movement brought together activists who answered these questions very differently. Mary Ware Dennett and Blanche Ames help us to see variability within the birth control movement, as well as its connections to the goals, debates, and strategies of reproductive health reform.

❦

Mary Ware Dennett (1872–1947) was born in Massachusetts into a respectable, entrenched New England family. Born Mary Coffin Ware to George Whitefield Ware and Livonia Coffin (Ames) Ware, Mary was the least privileged woman in this study. In complete contrast to Putnam, Dummer, and Ames, Mary's life was riddled with financial insecurities that began when her father, a wool merchant, died when she was ten years old. Upon her father's death, Dennett's mother moved her family to

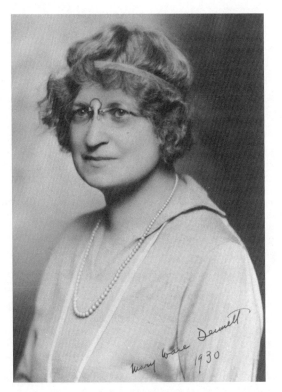

FIG. 3 MARY WARE DENNETT.
Photo courtesy of the Schlesinger Library, Radcliffe
Institute, Harvard University.

Boston, where Mary attended public school. In Boston, she began to spend significant amounts of time with her aunt, Lucia Ames Mead. A dedicated suffragist and pacifist, Aunt Lucia would inspire Mary's own activism in these two areas.

As a teenager, Dennett transferred to a private girls' high school in Northampton, Massachusetts. Miss Capen's School for Girls helped Mary develop not only her intellectual gifts, but also her appreciation and talent for art. After graduating, Dennett went on to study at the School of Art and Design at the Boston Museum of Fine Arts. In her early adulthood, it seemed that Dennett's life would revolve around her art. Before her thirtieth birthday, she had held a position in the Department of Design and Decoration at the Drexel Institute in Philadelphia, opened a handicraft shop with her sister in an attempt to master the lost art of leather design, and helped to organize the Boston Society of Arts and Crafts.

At age twenty-eight Mary Ware married Hartley Dennett, a Boston architect; the couple had two sons before their divorce in 1913.[1] The divorce motivated Mary to seek paid employment, as she had to support herself and her sons. Rather than relying on her art for income, Dennett found employment in various organizations devoted to social reform. Like Blanche Ames, Dennett's political activism began in the Massachusetts suffrage movement. She served as field secretary for the Massachusetts Woman Suffrage Association for two years and was then elected corresponding secretary of the National American Women's Suffrage Association (NAWSA) in 1910. By 1915 she branched out into other areas of reform, including the single tax and the antiwar movements.

When the United States entered World War I in 1917, Dennett protested by resigning as executive secretary of the Women's Section of the Democratic National Committee, and then joining numerous peace organizations including the People's Council, the Women's Peace Party, the Women's Peace Union, and the American Union Against Militarism. Dennett's involvement in the peace movement provided a unique and influential backdrop for her reproductive reform work, just as Dummer's attraction to German sex reformers and Putnam's conservative antistatism shaped their particular sensibilities about women, the state, and family life. It was the peace movement that first inspired Dennett's disdain for government repression, as the Wilson administration's treatment of dissenters was notorious for its harshness. This suspicion of state power and concern for civil liberties became the cornerstone of Dennett's political career.[2]

෴

Mary Ware Dennett's vision of the American birth control movement never quite coincided with that of the movement's powerful leader, Margaret Sanger. Lacking Sanger's charisma and almost ruthless compunction to lead, even Dennett's self-ascribed role as Sanger's rival has been challenged by historians of the birth control movement. It is certainly the case that Dennett achieved neither the fame nor the success of Margaret Sanger. However, Dennett's alternative vision and strategies lend an important context to Sanger's controversial career.

Throughout the interwar years, Dennett offered both a consistent critique of Sanger's tactics and ideology and served as an example of an alternative set of assumptions and strategies in the struggle for birth control. Her rivalry with Sanger was never as vicious as Putnam's with the Children's Bureau, nor quite as congenial as Dummer's gentle efforts to move the Bureau in new directions. As in the cases of Putnam and Dummer, however, Dennett's relations and disagreements with Sanger illuminate roads not taken in reproductive reform, and, more significantly, provide a context for understanding and evaluating how birth control strategies and policies were forged.[3]

Dennett's goal was to rescue birth control information from its legal and cultural association with obscenity. Her demands for freedom of information fell within a classically liberal political framework. In this way, Dennett managed to avoid a direct association with feminism, opting instead to ground her arguments in civil liberties. Despite her critics' assessment of her as politically naïve and unrealistic, Dennett consciously chose this political strategy for pragmatic reasons—it could simultaneously avoid the controversy associated with feminism and appeal to a deep-rooted cultural sentiment that valorized individualism and freedom from state regulation. In one sense, Dennett's tactics paralleled those of the progressive maternalists who used sentimental rhetoric and appealed to the sanctity of motherhood while pushing for innovative public health initiatives and policies; both Dennett and the women in the Children's Bureau tried to capitalize on traditional values in order to advance progressive causes. Dennett, however, misjudged the resistance she would face in her struggle to infuse the discourses of democracy and freedom with the controversial issue of sexuality.[4]

Eschewing maternalism, feminism, and "welfarism," Dennett's liberalism exposes another strategic option for reproductive reformers. Her stated goals were never to lower maternal and infant mortality rates or to free women from the procreative aspects of sexuality. Dennett sought, instead, to promote access to birth control information and materials as an expression of American women's fundamental right to get all necessary information about their health and bodies. For her, the problems of motherhood stemmed from ignorance and a heavy-handed and inappropriate state censorship apparatus. Where maternalists and feminists honed in on women's suffering and women's rights respectively, Dennett's liberalism targeted more universal concepts such as democratic access to information and the setting of reasonable limits for state power. Thus, like those of Putnam and Dummer, Dennett's career furthers our exploration of the political diversity that constituted reproductive reform activism in the interwar years. At this critical juncture in women's political history, Dennett's choices show that alternatives to maternalism and feminism did not necessarily yield better results.

This chapter will trace Dennett's work in the birth control movement, focusing on her relationship to Sanger in an effort to clarify the extent of their philosophical and political differences. I will show that, unlike Sanger's, Dennett's agenda and goals remained relatively consistent over time. This consistency stemmed from a principled and stubborn right-eousness that was at once her most admirable quality as a political reformer and a major reason for her political failures.

DENNETT, SANGER, AND THE ORIGINS OF THE NATIONAL BIRTH CONTROL LEAGUE

In Margaret Sanger's autobiography, the first glimpse we get of Mary Dennett is on the occasion of Sanger's return from Europe in 1915. Sanger implies that the National Birth Control League (NBCL) had been purposely reorganized during her absence and taken over by Dennett and others, who somehow managed to obtain Sanger's files and her list of subscribers to the *Woman Rebel*.[5] Sanger appealed to the new leadership of the NBCL for support during her upcoming trial; she reports that these well-heeled ladies politely disapproved of "my methods, my tactics, with everything I had done."[6] Presumably, the NBCL aimed to reform the laws regarding birth control "in an orderly and proper manner," and therefore could not countenance Sanger's civil disobedience. Here Sanger first began to paint a picture of Dennett and her group as politically timid and less than scrupulous. Furthermore, Sanger criticized Dennett's efforts to associate with "socially prominent and distinguished persons" to promote the cause. This accusation has contributed to Dennett's reputation for eschewing radicals and radical politics. Some historians promoted this conception of Dennett and interpreted her lack of socialist political commitment as a measure of her overall political incompetence or merely superficial dedication to women's rights.[7,8] However, Dennett represented the vast majority of white middle-class women reformers in the interwar years whose political origins lay in the suffrage fight, not in the labor struggle.

Dennett's interpretation of the early days of the movement diverged sharply from Sanger's. Indeed, far from pushing Sanger out, Dennett recalled asking her to serve on the executive committee of the NBCL upon her return from Europe. However, Dennett was rebuked. She explained that Sanger "felt it to be her particular function to break the laws rather than to spend effort at that time trying to change them."[9] In her own book, *Birth Control Laws,* published in 1926, Dennett gave Sanger proper credit for "touch(ing) off the spark that flamed into what has been called . . . the American birth control movement."[10] Continuing with this metaphor, she recalled, with some distaste, the agitational origins of the birth control movement, describing it as having "burst into flame about ten years ago with a sensational campaign to induce defiance of the laws on a large scale."[11] She cited Sanger's brazen editorials in her earliest periodical, the *Woman Rebel*, claiming that these tirades set the movement back even as they began it. Dennett did hope to reform the laws in an "orderly and proper manner," or, as she put it, in a "quiet business-like" way.[12] She argued that "assailing and defying the laws without taking steps to change them, naturally induced a more dramatic situation" than was necessary and only served to alienate politicians.[13] While Sanger's early propaganda cultivated the idea that "the struggle was bound to be a very long and bitter one," Dennett initiated a positive political effort.[14] Thus, from the very beginning of their rocky relationship, Sanger and Dennett illustrated different political temperaments, if not goals.

When Sanger met Dennett upon her return from Europe in 1915, Dennett had accomplished much more in her political life than merely organizing the NBCL. An artisan by vocation, Dennett was also an ardent suffragist and peace activist. She served as the field secretary of the Massachusetts Woman Suffrage Association from 1908 to 1910, during which time her achievements and organizational skills caught the attention of the women in the NAWSA. In the spring of 1910 Dennett was offered a job as corresponding secretary of the NAWSA. This position brought Dennett to New York City where, like Sanger, she met and became attracted to a wide array of social reformers and political causes.[15]

Prior to her move to the city, Dennett's main interest lay in the arts and crafts movement. Inspired by English architects and artisans, the arts and crafts movement envisioned a world in which beauty mattered and individuals worked to create functional and beautiful objects. The movement was about more than mere aesthetics; Dennett was attracted to its inherent critique of industrial capitalism. Similarly, Dennett's early interest in Henry George's single tax movement stemmed from her belief that it represented "a great fundamental social idea, rather than . . . a fiscal reform."[16]

Dennett was no revolutionary, but, like many progressives, she firmly believed in social transformation. In fact, Dennett's decision to leave the NAWSA in 1914 sprang from her disappointment in the narrowness, timidity, and tumult she perceived as strangling the suffrage movement. Only two years into the job at the NAWSA, Dennett wrote to president Anna Howard Shaw that suffrage was, "just a bore unless it is on a background of big inspiring progressive and fundamentally important work."[17] This sentiment, and Dennett's other reform causes, reveal a much more complex figure than the one Sanger caricatured in her autobiography.

Frustration with the NAWSA did not dampen Dennett's reform spirit as she soaked in a variety of political views and lifestyles in New York City's Greenwich Village. Among the reformers and radicals she associated with were the radical feminists of Heterodoxy, an intriguing group of women that included Katharine Anthony, Charlotte Perkins Gilman, Mabel Dodge, Crystal Eastman, Elizabeth Gurley Flynn, and Rose Pastor Stokes. Although loath to self-identify as a feminist (let alone a radical feminist), Dennett was nevertheless open-minded, attracted to new ideas, and committed to making the world a more humane and beautiful place.

Membership in the Intercollegiate Socialist Society and involvement in various progressive causes during her years in New York City launched her into the movement that would connect her suffrage and birth control activities and provide a strong ideological fulcrum for her subsequent political career. From 1914 on, Dennett, like many progressives, dedicated herself to keeping the United States out of the European war.

After resigning from the NAWSA, Dennett became the field secretary for the American Union Against Militarism (AUAM). Founded by Lillian Wald (its first president), Jane Addams, and Florence Kelley, the AUAM worked against preparedness and for mediation by neutrals to end the European conflict. Dennett was hired as a "prize agitator" to organize mass meetings. She agreed to work for Wilson's reelection in 1916 based on his pledge to keep the United States out of the war, and then resigned from the women's section of the Democratic National Committee when he reneged on this promise. Entrance into World War I prompted Dennett to make work for peace a priority. However, her experiences as an antiwar activist led her to other causes that would become new priorities. Illustrating her comfort with a wide range of political arenas, she became active in both the middle-class, maternalist Women's Peace Party and the radical People's Council of America.[18]

The mistreatment of pacifists by the Wilson administration during the war has been well documented. Subject to censorship, indictment, and incarceration, the AUAM formed a Civil Liberties Bureau in June 1917 to combat this treatment. By the fall, the Civil Liberties Bureau separated from the AUAM to become the autonomous National Civil Liberties Bureau—the precursor to the American Civil Liberties Union. Working within these pacifist organizations, Dennett initiated a lifelong involvement in the civil liberties movement that would shape her perspective on and activism in the arena of birth control, ultimately keeping her out of the mainstream.[19] Her background reveals that her commitment to birth control evolved out of a deeply felt commitment to women's rights, peace, and social justice, regardless of whether she consciously decided to market her birth control activities as part and parcel of these other movements.

ofo

Despite Dennett's and Sanger's total failure to cooperate in the early years, Dennett and Sanger made initial efforts that were, nonetheless, far less distinctive than they would later become. From 1917 to 1919, Dennett's NBCL dedicated itself to lobbying the state legislature of New York at Albany for the removal of contraception from the obscenity laws. Like Sanger, Dennett had yet to be convinced that sidestepping state legislatures in favor of federal reform was the most efficient political strategy. In this early period, Sanger and Dennett shared the belief that birth control should be fought for as an issue of free speech. Thus, the two issues that would come to separate them and upon which they would build separate organizations and distinct power bases had at this point not yet materialized.[20]

The NBCL's original goal was to galvanize public opinion in favor of birth control, but before long Dennett sought a more politically ambitious agenda. She felt relieved when the nine federal charges against Sanger were dropped in 1915. This seemed to Dennett to indicate that "the government itself did not deem the Comstock Laws in this regard, worth enforcing."[21] While Dennett embraced this positive sign of progress, negative experiences conspired to propel her into the federal arena. After three consecutive years of failure in Albany, she became frustrated with the New York State campaign. She came to believe that the federal Comstock Law was the precursor to all other birth control prohibitions. Thus, in 1919 she left the NBCL to launch the Voluntary Parenthood League (VPL), whose main ambition was reform of federal obscenity laws. In this endeavor, she sought to completely exempt birth control from obscenity prohibitions by repealing the offending sections of the law. By the time Dennett embarked on this new and ambitious campaign, however, Sanger had already disavowed the need for "clean repeal" in favor of a new "doctors-only" strategy, and the stage was set for years of competitive rivalry between the two women.

In 1918, Judge Crane of the New York State Court of Appeals affirmed the conviction of Sanger for selling contraceptive devices, but ruled that Section 1145 of the state obscenity code should not include physicians disseminating birth control for reasons of health. Sanger believed she had found the quickest and most pragmatic approach to birth control reform, and from then on worked exclusively for doctors-only legislation. She reasoned that if judges were willing to exclude doctors from obscenity prohibitions, then women could obtain birth control from their physicians. In her autobiography, Sanger argued that this change in strategy represented not just a pragmatic move, but a sincere ideological shift inspired by her trip to Europe in 1915. She remembers in her autobiography that her conversion to a belief in the necessity of medical regulation could be traced to visits to clinics in Holland and England, as well as discussions with one of her mentors, sexologist Havelock Ellis. She returned from Europe advocating the medically supervised dissemination of birth control information and articles. Dennett never believed this was the correct strategy for the movement to take and fought Sanger throughout the interwar years.

Dennett's resistance to medicalization ran counter not only to Sanger, but to the majority of reproductive health and rights activists in the interwar years. We have seen Putnam's unflinching faith in the medical profession to deliver reproductive health care services to women. But even the CB, which was castigated by Putnam for its emphasis on education over health care, sought to ally itself with physicians in order to promote preventive medicine and its prenatal care programs.[22] We will see in the next chapter that Ames also eagerly sought the cooperation of physicians to legitimate the birth control struggle in her home state. Dennett and Dummer, however, did not follow this path. For Dummer, physicians had little to do with the cultural oppression and its manifestation in the outmoded laws that she sought to eradicate. For Dennett, U.S. citizens deserved to have access to information without interference from a medical intermediary. Although arriving at their conclusions by different means, both Dummer and Dennett agreed that physicians did not hold out the best hope for ameliorating the problems of motherhood.

The decision of whether to cooperate with physicians or to emphasize the health aspects of reproductive reform was clearly based on strategic as well as ideological considerations. Indeed, this study has attempted to discern the variety of factors—both internal and external—that shaped the decisions of reformers. In the case of the birth control movement, reformers clearly understood the radical implications of their cause, but sought to cloak this potential in different ways. While Sanger's strategy involved transforming advocacy for birth control from a fight for social justice into a medical issue, Dennett had her own ideas about how to disassociate birth control reform from radicalism. She steered clear of direct association with Sanger, the creation of clinics, and the rhetoric of both feminism and the labor struggle. Dennett sought, rather, to connect birth control with rationality, democracy, and personal freedom—what she would one day characterize as "Constitutionally guaranteed old-fashioned American liberty."[23] Claiming that birth control was as unnatural as "toothbrushes, forks, knives, and agriculture,"[24] Dennett emphasized its links to civility and progress (and thus to humanity, rather than to women per se).

For Dennett, the only logical means of attaining the freedom and self-determination she sought was through legislation that would remove all references to birth control from the federal Comstock Laws. She reasoned that birth control information had been "mistakenly" classified as obscenity in 1873, setting an unfortunate precedent for states to follow. Therefore, federal reform would bring about the quickest remedy for "human suffering and ignorance."[25] She argued that, "[s]tate legislation without Federal action . . . is hardhearted and unintelligent; why break down the barriers to information slowly a state or two at a time and keep struggling worried parents in all the other states waiting for the information much of which they might have quickly by the passage of a Federal bill?"[26] Dennett's faith in federal action surely developed from her experience in the women's suffrage movement, which also moved from the state to the federal arena in the wake of several state referenda losses in the teens. In fact, she was a supporter of Alice Paul's efforts to revitalize the suffrage movement around a federal constitutional amendment, even if she disapproved of Paul's more militant tactics.[27] This orientation, which eschewed militant tactics while striving for substantial political goals, would characterize Dennett's entire career. Significantly, Dennett here contrasted sharply with Sanger, who in this period engaged in more outlandish behavior but did not regard federal reform as viable. Several years later, Sanger would come to conclusions that were similar to Dennett's and would work to tone down and clean up her rhetoric in order to make birth control accessible to the greatest possible number of women.

By 1919, Dennett's convictions led her to leave the NBCL to form a new organization dedicated specifically to federal reform. Her letter of resignation as secretary of the NBCL explained, "I am one of the three people who founded the League in 1915 . . . who believe that the time is fully ripe for successful work. I therefore do not want to remain a member of a Committee which does not feel equal to undertaking anything besides volunteer efforts."[28] Once again, as was the case with her departure from the NAWSA, Dennett chose to leave an organization whose political goals were too timid. She believed that purely educational work had become passé and that the time was ripe for political action. Dennett's move from a voluntary association to a full-fledged political lobbying organization anticipated a larger trend among women reformers in the postsuffrage decades. According to historian Michael McGerr, men's and women's political styles would basically converge by the 1920s. Women abandoned the radicalism and separatism associated with the last decade of the suffrage struggle in favor of a self-interested political style that depended on lobbying to accomplish their goals.[29] In this context, Dennett's (and then later, Sanger's) lack of success as a lobbyist reflects not merely a personal failure, but the ambiguous and contested consequences of women's entrance into the formal political sphere.[30]

THE VPL AND THE FEDERAL CAMPAIGN

In 1919, Dennett embarked on an ambitious campaign to convince the U.S. Congress that individual freedom should and must include a woman's freedom to information regarding her own and her family's health and welfare. In many ways, Dennett's sense of timing could not have been better. Women were about to be enfranchised by the Nineteenth Amendment, insuring them the most basic of all rights in a democratic republic. In addition, Dennett's campaign could also benefit from wartime concerns about infant and maternal welfare, public health, and family life. This would seem to have been a logical time for birth control reformers to ask for access to information that would allow women's dual roles as citizens and mothers to be both safer and more meaningful.

Dennett's formal introduction to the political process began with her visits to Washington, D.C., in 1919 to interview politicians for sponsorship of her "clean repeal" or "open" birth control bill. She called her bill by these names to highlight her differences from Sanger. However, only those in birth control circles would have been likely to care about or comprehend these distinctions, as Sanger had yet to embark on her rival federal campaign.

Dennett was met by prejudice and allusive tactics in Washington. Despite her conviction that, by 1919, the time was ripe for federal birth control reform, the vast majority of Americans, including elected officials, were uncomfortable with the subject to the point of being unwilling to even discuss it. On the eve of dramatic changes in the nation's mores regarding sexuality, birth control was still considered an offensive or obscene topic, certainly one that did not belong in the arena of national politics. Indeed, as we have seen, Putnam and her antisuffrage allies had been fabricating an association between suffrage and birth control in order to malign the former movement.

As suffragists fought for the integrity of their movement, maternal and infant welfare activists in the CB decried any association with birth control. They had learned to fight for programs and privileges on the basis of the sanctity of motherhood and the family. Consequently, they took great pains to position birth control outside the parameters of legitimate programs and policies. This strategy was necessary to achieve the passage of the Sheppard-Towner Act in 1921. Political support for Sheppard-Towner continued to be at least partially predicated on its distance from the birth control movement throughout the 1920s.[31] Dennett, however, never identified as a maternalist and did not accept birth control as a liability. In the face of resistance and outright rejection from mainstream politicians as well as many within reproductive reform circles, Dennett adopted strategies that, in retrospect, were creative and principled but unsuccessful.

While Dennett's political style was more cautious than Sanger's in the late teens and early twenties, her tactics were more ambitious. These differences in approach stemmed from personal temperament as well as Dennett's earlier and more direct engagement in the political process. While Dennett spent her days interviewing legislators, Sanger was using the language of both feminism and socialism to stir up public sentiment. For example, in the January 1920 issue of the *Birth Control Review* (*BCR*) the headlines on the front cover and the leading editorial, written by Sanger, recommended, "A Birth Strike to Avert World Famine."[32] Dennett reacted strongly to this editorial, charging that the movement's "progress is seriously menaced by injecting into the situation a militantly feministic policy or the terminology of the labor struggle."[33] She cogently argued, "It is obvious that the majority of Congressmen are not warm hearted toward the [birth] strike idea in general, and neither are they moved by feminism. On the contrary, they are antagonized by both. But they are reasonably hospitable to all the basic reasons for passing the bill; public health, child welfare, the lessening of the need for charity, decreased public expenditures for the care of the unfit, increased industrial stability, etc."[34] Thus, Dennett recognized the futility of pitching birth control as a means toward women's emancipation or economic justice years before Sanger would come to this same conclusion. However, even when Sanger decided to drop the offending rhetoric, she moved in different directions than did Dennett.

Dennett found the propaganda of the *BCR* damaging to the cause because it antagonized the very politicians who were instrumental to initiating and sustaining legislative reform. However, Sanger was not yet trying to reform federal law in this period. Her main interests lay in establishing clinics and public education through propaganda and civil disobedience. Therefore, she found it unnecessary to placate congressmen.

Dennett shied away from rhetoric and propaganda that would alienate legislators, and decided to resign from the board of directors of the *BCR* over the editorial. Although she assured board members that she would be "heartily glad to continue any informal conferences . . . in any way which will help the cause," she did not want her federal lobbying efforts threatened by her association with explosive issues and controversial propaganda.[35] But Dennett's objections to Sanger were more than pragmatic. Dennett sincerely believed that, while Sanger was intent on breaking laws and humiliating legislators, *she* would be the one to successfully reform the laws that kept contraceptive information out of the hands of American women and men.

Dennett used various tactics to make the movement more palatable to politicians. Her principal political contribution lay in stressing its implications for civil liberties and freedom of speech, press, and information. In her attempts to gain political acceptance, however, she miscalculated the power of classical liberal thought, underestimating deep resistance to the inclusion of women, mothers, and issues of sexuality in arguments for liberty, justice, and individualism. One way to understand this particular miscalculation is as a reflection of women's historically ambiguous citizenship status. As Carole Pateman and others have argued, women's motherhood role has contributed to their economic and political disadvantage. According to T. H. Marshall, "those who have only restricted access to economic participation are implicitly denied a portion of their rights as citizens."[36] Dennett's claims therefore missed their mark, for the rights and responsibilities of citizenship had never been fully granted to women. Thus, her discourse, while intended to be familiar, patriotic, and even comforting, did not relay the powerful message she hoped it would. On a more practical level, Dennett did not invoke the cooperation of what would become the most significant interest group involved in the cause, namely, the American Medical Association (AMA). Ultimately, her decisions to subvert medical authority and to make her appeal on the basis of human rights and individual freedom cost Dennett the broad-based support necessary to sustain a successful political campaign. She would ultimately come to discover what Sanger and many others in the movement had already guessed: that birth control would flounder without the sanitizing effect of an alignment with physicians.[37]

Although Dennett's decision to fight for a comprehensive reform bill that would exempt contraception from the category of obscenity might have seemed to her a logical, principled, and efficient way to promote birth control, this approach was clearly reprehensible to the medical community. She liked to think that physicians would just as readily support her "open bill" as they would a doctors-only bill; this assumption did not turn out to be well founded. After Judge Crane's decision in Sanger's 1918 trial, physicians generally agreed that state laws would be interpreted so as to exempt physicians from obscenity prohibitions. Therefore, many physicians interpreted Dennett's federal efforts as either unnecessary or potentially threatening to their professional rights. The New York Academy of Medicine, for example, told Dennett that it had no interest in supporting her legislative efforts, which it condemned for promoting "indiscriminate distribution" of birth control information and materials.[38] For her part, Dennett challenged physicians to support legislation that they disinterestedly believed would most effectively reduce death, disease, and suffering. In her 1921 pamphlet "The Laws Against Contraceptive Knowledge," she argued that, "[T]he whole profession, in justice to itself, should hasten to support the broad legislation which will free it from any possible suggestion that the medical point of view is not one of disinterested readiness to meet human needs and to prevent suffering to the greatest possible degree."[39]

Not surprisingly, the organized medical community never accepted this more liberal birth control bill, which would have sidestepped medical authority over information and distribution. By the 1920s the AMA had devoted considerable effort to professionalizing, eliminating quacks and "irregulars," and tightening control over medical training and practice. Physicians had begun to crack down on thinly veiled advertisements for contraceptives, abortifacients, and abortion services, all of which were illegal, presumably dangerous to women's health, and unregulated. Therefore, many physicians were anxious about the "indiscriminate distribution" of the information and materials that Dennett seemed to be advocating.

Lacking the approval of the medical community, Dennett searched for prominent individuals to lend their reputation to the movement. As we have seen, Elizabeth Putnam was one of the prominent citizens Dennett sought out for endorsement in 1919.[40] Dennett asked Putnam to envision how access to "this much needed information on sex hygiene" would increase human health and happiness. Putnam never responded, although she might have been more comfortable in Dennett's movement than she would have guessed, as it distinguished itself in reproductive reform circles by its distaste for excessive government regulation. When Dennett arrived in Washington, D.C., on behalf of the VPL, she was determined to educate congressmen and to find supporters who would risk introducing her measure. The VPL purposely steered clear of publicity and public propaganda campaigns during the first two years of its efforts in Washington. In this way, it tried to distinguish itself from Sanger's antagonistic style. While the VPL prided itself on developing a good rapport with legislators, Sanger's *BCR* was concurrently carrying headlines that read, "WANTED: INTELLIGENCE TESTS FOR LEGISLATORS."[41] In this editorial piece, Sanger boldly proclaimed that, "A State Legislature represents the last bulwark of prejudice, superstition, and ignorance." She singled out the Codes Committee of the New York State Legislature, calling it "a small group of adolescent minds."[42] The VPL's *Birth Control Herald* (*BCH*), on the other hand, offered a more positive interpretation of its own frustrating political predicament, arguing that the Congressmen who are responsible for repealing the objectionable sections of the Comstock Law, "will be blessed by millions."[43] Even years later, Dennett argued that the average legislator "did not in any way live up to the picture of an 'oppressive force.'"[44] Her generosity toward legislators certainly grew out of her determination to proceed with legislative reform. She eschewed agitational propaganda in favor of a political strategy that was simultaneously more personal and professional than Sanger's; she sought interviews with individual congressmen while formally lobbying for a clean repeal bill.

Dennett found that it was much easier to find private supporters of her open bill than it was to find public endorsers or sponsors. Her campaign diaries from this period record her continual disappointment with politicians who refused to take a public stand on this controversial issue. One of the first congressmen she sought out was Senator Morris Sheppard (D-Texas) who would soon sponsor the innovative and controversial Sheppard-Towner Act of 1921. Dennett referred to Sheppard in her diary as "another friend made," but one who would not commit to sponsorship until his own maternity bill was passed.[45] Dennett could not find a sponsor until January 1923, when Senator Albert B. Cummins (R-Iowa) agreed to introduce a bill on behalf of the VPL.

Dennett faced opposition not only from timid and hostile congressmen in her lobbying campaign of 1920, but also from those within the birth control movement. In that same year, as Dennett searched for a sponsor, Sanger gave the first in a long line of speeches that denied that there was rivalry in the movement and asserted her own authority. According to Dennett, Sanger "trotted out that New York doctors and nurses bill, as if it were the center of an internationally supported organization, slurred over the federal law as a trifling matter,—and outlined a program of *state*-action that would last till Kingdom come. No mention of the VPL whatever,—isn't life queer?"[46]

In 1921, after Dennett had spent two years in Washington trying unsuccessfully to secure a sponsor for her bill, Sanger formed the American Birth Control League (ABCL). Her league committed itself to the establishment of clinics and, for this purpose, sought doctors-only legislation on the state level. Dennett worried that the new league would seek to discredit the type of birth control bill advocated by the VPL. Although never overtly oppositional (in that the ABCL did not concern itself with federal legislation at the time), Dennett harbored resentment over the mere existence of the meddling ABCL. She feared that two painstaking years of political work would be undermined by an organization led by Sanger. The two women regarded each other as sincere yet fundamentally misguided and, therefore, as a threat to the movement of which each claimed leadership. Dennett argued that the ABCL's antagonism to the VPL and its goals "was obvious from the statement of the leaders, the refusal to cooperate and from various editorials in the *BCR*."[47]

By the end of the year, it was clear that Sanger and Dennett could not reach a compromise. Their rivalry took on its overt characteristics: Dennett resigned from the board of directors of the *BCR*, Sanger introduced a doctors-only bill in the New York State legislature, and, in November, Dennett was purposely silenced at the first American Birth Control Conference. Sanger did not allow Dennett to present her paper at the conference precisely because Dennett had prepared a speech on the virtues of the VPL's political strategy as compared to the faulty logic displayed by the ABCL and the Sanger wing of the movement. Dennett had planned to argue before the entire reform community that changing the federal law against providing birth control information would be the most efficient and pragmatic way for the birth control movement to proceed in the 1920s. Part of her speech read, "Obviously . . . the most far-reaching single step to be taken in changing this mass of repressive laws is to revise the Federal law first . . . which is not only effective in itself, but which serves as a most powerful example for the States to follow. This is the key to the whole situation."[48] Sanger, who wished to appear as the one and only leader of an already precarious movement, regarded Dennett's prepared speech as a threat to the cause and to her personal authority. Each woman believed she possessed a more savvy level of understanding of the complex political obstacles to the legalization of birth control.

Prior to 1924, when Sanger announced her intention to begin working in the federal arena, Dennett could hope that the birth control movement would proceed along two ideological and tactical lines—with Sanger working on doctors-only legislation at the state level, and the VPL working for clean repeal at the federal level. In 1923 the *BCH* reported, "The VPL is not working against Mrs. Sanger, . . . there is room in the field for more than one group, but . . . we believe our program to be the broader and the quicker and therefore the one that should be achieved first.[49] Dennett was so convinced of the wisdom of her tactics that she asked only that Sanger stay out of her way and allow her to get the job done, quickly and quietly.

Dennett found sponsors for the VPL's bill by the end of 1922. She claimed that the League's desire for action, rather than publicity, had led to its initial success. Senator Cummins and Representative John Kissel of the Third District of New York (Brooklyn) introduced the VPL's bill "to rectify Comstock" on January 10, 1923. The bill (Senate Bill No. S4314 and House Bill No. HR13756) would have removed the words "preventing contraception" from Sections 211 and 245 of the Criminal Code and from Sections 102, 312, and 305 of the Tariff Act of 1922.

Disappointment gripped the VPL as the last session of the Sixty-Seventh Congress came to a close without any action taken on the Cummins-Kissel Bill. According to *BCH* headlines, the bill "had enough probable votes for favorable report in Senate Judiciary and Sub-Committee of House."[50] It was clear now to the members of the VPL that merely securing a sponsor would not ensure success. The VPL was a newcomer to the lobbying and legislative process and did not accurately assess the significance of its bill in relation to the other business of Congress. In the 1923 Congressional Report in the *BCH*, women reformers described what they perceived as a somewhat haphazard and baffling process—"Battling against time and the accidents of illness and the embarrassment of Senators—. . . the bill had been submerged along with 14,000 other bills."[51]

The Congress took no action on the bill and, by the next year, Representative Kissel had dropped out of the fight. In January 1924, Cummins introduced the bill in the Senate and Representative William Vaile of Colorado introduced the bill in the House. A number of prominent citizens attended the Cummins-Vaile Bill hearings. According to Dennett, Roman Catholics swelled the ranks of the opposition. Dennett's *Birth Control Laws* recounts highlights of testimony during the hearings, with a special focus on the position against Catholic interference with free speech articulated by Dorothy Glases, the wife of a professor of biology at Amherst College. Glases argued against the Catholic position with an analogy.

> Suppose, gentlemen, that the Christian Scientists came to you and said that they could not keep their people from using doctors. Would you then pass legislation to do away with medical knowledge at the request of the Christian Scientists? We have no objection to their taking any attitude on this matter, but we do object to their method of forcing it on others. We wish to be free to create scientific values without their interference.[52]

This argument was heard over and over in efforts to promote the open bill. Dennett and her followers pitted the virtues of scientific freedom against the threat of parochial ignorance.

After its first bill was buried, the VPL looked forward with optimism to the opening of the next session of Congress in 1924. Before the last session had ended, Senator Cummins promised to reintroduce the bill and, according to *BCH* headlines, predicted, "Next Time You Will Win."[53] But the next session provided no opportunities; the VPL entered a period of gradual collapse. Characterized by growing disappointment over the congressional response, 1924 was also the year Sanger announced that she herself would begin working on federal legislative reform. Of course, her bill would follow the course that she had charted on the state level, asking only for medical exemptions from birth control prohibitions.

Sanger's 1924 announcement placed the ABCL's program in more direct conflict with the VPL than was the case when the latter organization had been the sole birth control group lobbying Congress. Whereas five frustrating years in Washington, D.C., had deflated the VPL's optimism, Sanger's popularity was growing as she moved away from her radical origins in favor of an alliance with the organized medical community. Sanger's willingness—even desire—to be in the public eye had engendered the publicity that Dennett avoided but that naturally brought money with it. The VPL now faced a formidable, well-financed rival. Dennett, however, did not give up entirely her fight for what she considered a more comprehensive reform bill. She continued in her efforts to convince fellow reformers, politicians, the general public, and even physicians that straight repeal made more sense and was infinitely more just.

⚛

Once Sanger decided to move into the federal arena in the mid-1920s, she assumed that Dennett and her bothersome VPL would move aside to accommodate her political agenda and tactics. The ABCL even went so far as to approach Senator Cummins and Representative Vaile, the congressmen for whom the VPL's bill was named, to present them with an amendment to the bill that would transform it into doctors-only legislation. The legislative secretary of the ABCL, Ann Kennedy, wrote to the members of the VPL to inform them of her organization's intentions, implying that VPL opposition would only harm the cause, as the ABCL's strategy was infinitely more practical. According to Kennedy, even Cummins and Vaile themselves agreed that the ABCL's amendment to the original bill "would eliminate much of the objection raised."[54] Kennedy continued her letter in a polite tone that barely masked the direct challenge she was offering to the VPL's federal legislative lobbying program. "Our Congressional work will proceed along these lines and as a believer in birth control and interested in federal work, we would appreciate your cooperation in this field."[55]

Dennett, however, would not back down in the face of the ABCL, despite its organizational and financial superiority and its national connections. Dennett wrote to Senator Cummins to warn him of the encroaching ABCL.

> I am quite certain that you will be urged by the birth control group of which Margaret Sanger is president . . . to alter your bill and to compromise on the principles on which your bill is based. I most earnestly hope it will be impossible to persuade you to compromise. I am determined to retain my confidence that you will continue to believe . . . that genuine freedom is worth securing and preserving.[56]

Dennett attempted to play hardball with the Sangerists, for she felt that the activities of the ABCL placed her in an impossible situation in which she had to defend the logic of her original bill against an assault by the largest and most prestigious birth control organization in the United States. In a letter to Cummins urging him to maintain his commitment to "genuine freedom," Dennett admitted that she had "said very little . . . in the past about the work of Mrs. Sanger and her organization."[57] Although Dennett acknowledged that Sanger had "done a great deal of good" for the cause, she advised Cummins that, in dealing with the VPL, he was associating with the oldest and most experienced birth control league in the country in regard to federal legislative reform. In contrast, Sanger's "interest in legislation is very recent and her organization is a relatively new one. It is only a little over two years old."[58] Dennett then went on to explain how Sanger and her group might appear more powerful or experienced than they really were. "[O]wing to Mrs. Sanger's wide, personal reputation, her new organization has had a great deal more money given to it than we have had. The publicity work that has thus been made possible has made a great many people take it for granted that Mrs. Sanger has great legislative wisdom as well as persistent interest in this cause."[59] Dennett ended her letter to Senator Cummins with a subtle warning. She asked him to consider only what would make the best legislation in the long run, and not to play politics with personal freedom. Imploring him to carefully consider his accountability for the choices he made, she wrote, "I don't want Americans to wake up a few years from now and find that the laws on this subject which they helped to have passed, are basically wrong and inadequate."[60]

By the mid-1920s, as their activities began to directly infringe upon each other, Sanger and Dennett became less than cordial toward each other. In addition to becoming aware of ideological and political differences regarding the course of the movement, Dennett began to wince under Sanger's increasingly tight control of public relations and propaganda. In 1925, Dennett once again faced censorship by Sanger, as the latter barred full representation of the VPL at the sixth International Birth Control Conference in New York. Sonia Bronson, secretary of the VPL, described this unfortunate situation in a letter to Dennett suggesting that the prominent Rabbi Stephen Wise might speak on behalf of the VPL.

> They . . . asked him to bring up this matter of Mrs. Sanger ignoring the work of the VPL so shamefully, and raise a delegation right then and there to have the work of this league fully represented at the conference. It seems to me the best opportunity for putting before the public . . . Mrs. Sanger's attitude, and asking them to demand fair play. Something drastic should be done. It's ridiculous to let her play the game any which way she chooses, so long as she amuses herself.[61]

Bronson was concerned not only with Sanger's underhanded tactics, but also with her virtual monopoly over public education campaigns for birth control, which she felt left the general public and the reform community with a skewed picture. We get a sense of her frustration when she writes, "When I think of Mrs. Sanger and think of how she leads them all around by the nose, some of the wisest as well as the stupidest, I am overwhelmed, appalled."[62]

In the spring of 1925, the VPL initiated a conference to promote cooperation between itself, the ABCL, and Dr. Robert L. Dickinson's New York–based Committee on Maternal Health (CMH). Dennett realized that her VPL was clearly in a weak position and needed to make a gesture to its competition. Neither the ABCL nor the CMH agreed to participate in this effort to reach common ground, although Dennett did meet with unofficial representatives from each group.[63] According to Dennett's report of the informal discussion that took place, both the ABCL and the CMH had members who were in favor of liberalizing the positions of their respective organizations with regard to the dissemination of birth control information. In spite of its ultimate failure to encourage consensus, the meeting was an opportunity for the VPL to make suggestions to members of the other two groups. For example, the minutes record a suggestion that a birth control bill incorporating demands from all sides might allow not only doctors, but also legitimate businesses, to mail contraceptive information and technology. Another issue the VPL raised was the precarious status of nurses and social workers under a doc-tors-only-type law.[64] Dennett clearly realized that, despite her legitimate claim to be the undisputed pioneer in the arena of federal birth control legislation, she could not afford to rest on her laurels in an increasingly competitive political atmosphere. The fact that both the ABCL and the CMH could refuse to participate in the conference initiated by the VPL reflected the uneven balance of power that had developed among the three groups.

Dennett stopped lobbying and resigned as president of the VPL in the spring of 1925. She now became the Consultative Chair of the VPL's National Council. Faltering in the face of its rivals, Dennett's VPL looked for new ways to bring its message to legislators and the general public. Sonia Bronson suggested to Dennett that she write a book on the history of birth control laws in the United States, analyzing revisions and amendments, and making "a plea for the support of laws which are sound, enforceable, and efficacious."[65] Dennett agreed that, due to Sanger's latest interest in federal legislation, the time had come "when it is peculiarly worth while to help the public to think clearly on this subject, so that the country may if possible be spared from fool legislation."[66] Dennett's concern was that time might be wasted on flawed legislation not worth fighting for. However, as Sanger would counter, practical steps taken in the right direction would facilitate dissemination of birth control through medically supervised clinics. Ironi-cally, this debate would become moot, as both women ultimately gave up on federal legislative reform as a viable strategy.

In 1926, Dennett published her first book, *Birth Control Laws: Shall We Keep Them, Change Them, or Abolish Them?*, in which she told her ver-sion of the history of the American birth control movement and made suggestions for its future. She traced the development of state laws back to the original Comstock Law and made a forceful case for an open bill. She presented a twofold argument, emphasizing both the practicality of, and the important principles supporting, the open bill. The book detailed Dennett's concerns about "struggling worried parents" and "the obvious fact that the ban on the circulation of knowledge . . . (was) . . . contrary to the right of freedom of the press."[67]

⊛

Once Sanger involved herself with federal reform, the VPL's authority in the field was undermined and its energies scattered in continual attempts to clarify its position in relation to the more visible Sangerists. The League found itself in the position of having to defend its existing claim to legislative reform, for Sanger's propaganda posited the VPL as the invading outsider who sought to split the movement through its advocacy of impractical legislation. Eventually, even VPL members began to doubt their own league's tactics, forcing the leadership to put out a memo defending itself.

> In pointing out to League members and friends the discrepancies in the doctors-only kind of legislation, we are only helping the public to be sure that it gets what it wants. . . . The ABCL knows as well as we do that there are countless families cut off from immediate medical service. What shall these mothers do? Shall we ask them to wait until they can save the necessary money it costs for them to travel to consult the nearest doctor.[68]

Thus, Sanger's visibility and powerful propaganda machine forced the VPL leadership to explain the disadvantages of the doctors-only strategy to its own members.

In addition to propaganda wars, the legislative battle continued between Sanger and the VPL. In 1926, Dennett sent careful instructions to Representative Vaile on how to handle Sanger.

> Your biggest chance for usefulness now . . . will be when Mrs. Sanger . . . gets someone to introduce the bill which they have announced. I think you can very quietly persuade the Committee to amend it by striking out everything after the enacting clause, and substituting your bill. Their bill as it stands is absurd. . . . The limitations which are provided are completely unenforceable . . . and aside from its futility as legislation . . . [it] merely permits a whole string of privileged people to do what would be an indecent crime if done by others who are not in the legally privileged class. A most un-American notion, is it not?[69]

Dennett's conviction that doctors-only legislation reflected the wrong path for the birth control movement to take—one that would be regretted for years to come—stemmed from an abstract yet strong sense of justice that simultaneously inspired unique, humane insights and blind spots in her perception.

IDEOLOGY, PRINCIPLE, AND THE QUESTION OF EUGENICS

The ways in which Dennett and Sanger interpreted the birth control issue had a great impact on their political styles and tactics. Whereas Sanger moved away from rhetoric lamenting the tyranny of government control over people's lives, Dennett steadfastly maintained this orientation throughout the interwar years. However, Dennett's critique of the federal laws did not stem from a radical or anarchist-inspired critique of the state. Rather, she worked for "a government that intends no oppression at home."[70] The alliance of Dennett's reform instincts with her aversion to state interference into people's lives facilitated and helps to explain, the trajectory of her career from activism in the areas of birth control, sex education, and, finally, free speech.

During the three years that Dennett spent in Washington on behalf of a VPL-sponsored birth control bill, she developed a comprehensive rationale for her federal reform and clean repeal strategies. In the pages of the *BCH*, readers were barraged with lists of reasons for favoring the Cummins-Kissel and then the Cummins-Vaile Bill, which were designed to be sent to senators and representatives. The basic reasons most frequently listed for support of such a bill included the following: people were already using birth control; birth control information was mistakenly classified as an obscenity under the Comstock Laws of 1873; birth control information was modern science, not indecency; the government had no right to suppress knowledge of any kind; the obscenity law was unenforceable; un-American tactics would be needed to enforce the federal ban on birth control information; and the reform bill facilitated access to information for those who sought it out without imposing that information on those who did not. These arguments were quite different from Sanger's and, indeed, most reproductive reformers; they downplayed issues of public health, ignored feminist perspectives, and eschewed the sentimental rhetoric of maternalism in favor of a more legalistic and constitutional framework.

Dennett and Sanger attempted to shape the movement in ways that reflected their overlapping, yet distinct, commitments and goals. For Sanger, the key issue was providing birth control to women. In order to accomplish this end, she tried to make sure physicians were reasonably knowledgeable about, and legally able and willing to prescribe, birth control to their patients. Thus, she divided her time between her particular kind of legislative reform, the establishment of clinics, and the fostering of medical research into contraceptive technologies. For her part, Dennett was less interested in how birth control would get into the hands of actual women than in the more abstract question of democratic access. In this sense, Dennett's agenda was similar to Putnam's in that the latter worked to clean up the milk supply for consumers rather than supply milk to poor mothers and babies. Whereas in Putnam's case this lack of interest in provision can be interpreted as indicative of a clear insensitivity to the poor and disadvantaged, Dennett's intentions are a bit more complicated. For instance, Dennett charged that Sanger's approach would not help poor women who lacked access to medical care. Like Putnam, however, Dennett's contributions to and perspective on reproductive reform were profoundly shaped by her larger political convictions.

Most of Dennett's arguments stemmed from a civil liberties foundation and were thus focused directly on the power of the federal government to interfere in the pursuit of knowledge, freedom, and happiness. Sanger, who early in her career as a reformer decried federal power over women's bodies, originally shared this line of argument. In the first issue of the *BCR*, for example, readers were asked to picture the government's "gaunt hand . . . reaching out its sinewy fingers over bench and bar."[71] Sanger, however, soon dropped this antagonistic stance; meanwhile, the VPL's *BCH* continued to ask "Has the government the right to keep knowledge away from people?" as it lobbied Congress in the 1920s.[72]

Dennett's formulation of the birth control issue reflected less interest in the problem of provision than did Sanger's. Sanger characterized this lack of interest as a great weakness in Dennett's perspective as well as in her legislation, arguing that, "[t]o offer a pamphlet to a woman who cannot read or who is too weary to understand its directions, is like offering a printed bill-of-fare to a starving man."[73] Sanger worried that "merely" opening up the mails would not insure women's ability to obtain information they could use and materials they needed. Dennett countered that, once it was no longer classified as obscene, birth control could be obtained through various means—at drug stores or from social workers—and that only exempting physicians would actually stifle the flow of information.[74]

The responses of Dennett and Sanger to letters asking for help reflect these different orientations. Sanger, ever the pragmatist, fought for doctors-only legislation and gave out birth control information to women who wrote to her for help, simultaneously breaking and working to change the law. Women who wrote to Dennett requesting information about contraception, received the same didactic response: "It is absolutely illegal to mail any contraceptive information anywhere in the country; and in many of our states . . . it is illegal to give the information by any means whatsoever. . . . Of course the laws are broken all the time. That is why it is time to repeal them. I hope you will help us accomplish it." Then Dennett undermined the strength of her own convictions by adding, "I hope you will get [the information] in spite of the laws. Have you asked your own physician?"[75] Here Dennett is admitting that physicians—at least until her reforms were successful—may indeed be the best group to provide contraceptive information to American women. However, she refused to bend in terms of her legislative agenda. Despite Sanger's comparatively commonsense approach, the appeals of needy women, and the obstacles on Capitol Hill, Dennett held out hope for her ultimate goal: complete repeal of the sections of the Comstock Laws that dealt with contraceptive information. It may be instructive at this point to recall Dummer's similar calls for total justice in the face of political and cultural obstacles. Just as Dennett wanted birth control information totally free from stigma, Dummer sought to rescue children born out of wedlock from any cultural, political, or economic disadvantage. Both women were loath to compromise their basic principles and decried what can now be seen in context as the more pragmatic approaches adopted by the mainstream.

Although Dennett's more abstract formulation of the birth control issue led her away from the problem of provision, it also prevented her from falling into the eugenic and racist framework that characterized the mainstream birth control movement in the interwar years. According to Carole McCann, eugenics served the movement in three major ways: it facilitated the framing of birth control as a public health issue, it linked it with the agenda of reproductive health reformers, and it helped mask the sexual nature of the cause.[76] McCann argues that, in spite of these political and rhetorical advantages, eugenics ultimately ended up "displacing women from the position of subjects of their own reproduction."[77] Most important for understanding Dennett's reaction to these trends, eugenics all but annihilates the individual. McCann writes, "Eugenicists were concerned with the social control of human reproduction; they had no concern that this control would be enacted on the bodies of women. In the language of population dynamics, the individual disappears entirely."[78] Dennett consistently maintained that the true beneficiaries of birth control reform would be individuals who would be able to obtain all the information they needed to make intelligent decisions and safeguard their own health and the health and welfare of their families. She warned fellow reformers against the tendency to forget the individual in favor of making grand claims for birth control as a social panacea.

Amidst growing concern in the 1920s about "race suicide," immigration restriction, miscegenation, and the manifestation of these concerns in forced sterilization legislation on the state level, Dennett steadfastly defended personal freedom. In a paper on "Birth Control, War and Population," she expressed alarm at a resolution passed at the neo-Malthusian conference held in London in 1922 that urged the League of Nations to call upon countries to "limit their populations to their own resources."[79] She noted that American birth control reformers had supported a similar program at the Disarmament Conference in Washington. Her salient objections deserve to be generously recounted:

> The idea in both instances seemed to be that governments as such were to secure this limitation by birth control. Just how governments were to enforce birth control was not indicated, but the mental picture which the idea creates is one of appalling paternalism, as well as a *shockingly unthinkable intrusion upon private life.* Governments may well assist in the spread of education as to the best methods for controlling conception, just as they now help to spread knowledge about raising crops and animals. *Giving people an opportunity to learn is a proper enough function for governments, but dictating to people as to how many children they shall have is . . . preposterous. . . .* this effort of the Neo-Malthusians and others to make governments act in some positive way is undoubtedly well meant . . . but it can hardly be considered the outcome of sound thinking.[80]

Dennett's critique articulated connections between international racism, totalitarianism, and imperialism. She pointedly warned against well-known and active eugenists, who appealed to fears "that the more prolific, undeveloped, unfit and dark-skinned peoples are sure to overwhelm the less prolific, highly civilized, more fit white skinned peoples."[81] Dennett urged that diverting attention to birth control for these reasons only served to mask the necessity of international social and economic reform. Accordingly, she argued that, "education and economic oppression are well worth worrying about in every country, but 'overpopulation' is not."[82]

In her opposition to state intervention and potential oppression in the arena of sexuality and motherhood, Dennett's arguments came closer to those of the anarchist, "free lover," and birth control pioneer Emma Goldman than they did to Margaret Sanger. Sensitive to the dangers of increased government intervention in private life, and to issues of class and race, Goldman fought for birth control because it would liberate women and sexuality. In a 1915 article on a plan to sterilize 15 million American "defectives," Goldman pointed out the potential dangers and ironies of sterilization and eugenic programs in a capitalist and racist society:

> [S]ince dear Mrs. Harriman, J. D. Rockefeller, A. G. Bell, Andrew Carnegie, Irving Fisher and so many other highly respectable folk are to finance this crusade, it is highly moral and 'eugenic.' It is hardly possible adequately to express one's admiration for these estimable people who are so certain of the defectiveness of numbers of the lower classes and so certain of their own godliness . . . [W]e modestly prefer to align ourselves with

whomever they choose to call defective, even at the risk of sterilization, rather than be placed in the same class with such holy eugenists.[83]

Although Dennett's own observations certainly lacked this biting class critique, she nevertheless correctly assessed the negative implications in the movement's turn away from individual rights and toward population control and sterilization in the United States and abroad. Dennett's failure to address the role of class led her to equate liberty and justice with individual rights rather than with government responsibility. Ironically, however, Dennett's focus on individual liberties kept her from supporting the increasingly racist rhetoric of the mainstream birth control movement.

The eugenic elements of mainstream birth control rhetoric connected the movement to sterilization activities in the 1920s and 1930s. The economic constraints of the Depression encouraged public acceptance of both contraception and sterilization. The 1930s also witnessed increased Catholic opposition to any kind of artificial limitation of family size and interference with natural reproductive functioning. Pope Pius's encyclical of 1930, "On Christian Marriage," condemned both practices, thereby bringing them closer together in a coherent political agenda, despite the opposition of individual birth control reformers to the eugenics movement.

Dennett's abhorrence of eugenics placed her at odds not only with Sanger and mainstream birth controllers, but also with such groups as the League of Women Voters, the American Association of University Women, and the General Federation of Women's Clubs (which supported sterilization laws in certain states).[84] By 1925 there were sterilization laws in seventeen states and, in the 1927 case *Buck v. Bell*, the Supreme Court ruled on the constitutionality of a Virginia sterilization law. This ruling bolstered the enactment and implementation of sterilization programs throughout the United States. Dennett had, from the beginning of her involvement in the movement, challenged limitations placed on personal freedom. Her orientation offered a way for her to critique the two main trends of the birth control movement in the interwar years: the medicalization of the movement, and the tendency to argue for the social, not the individual, benefits of birth control.

☙❧

Throughout the 1920s, Sanger and Dennett became increasingly familiar with the legislative process. Ironically, despite these women's political jockeying, the movement would attain its earliest victories through the judicial, rather than the legislative, branch of government. Even late into the 1920s and through the 1930s, Congress posed a dead end for the birth control movement. In January 1926, for example, one of the politicians who had initially pledged to introduce the VPL's bill politely announced that he would refrain from introducing it in the present session of Congress. He argued that, "there is no possibility whatsoever of its passage or even its favorable report by the judiciary committee of either House. . . . There must be more of a public demand for it before it will have even a fighting chance in Congress, and the development of such demand must be done on the outside, not the inside, of the national legislature."[85]

After lobbying for over six years (battling Sanger head-on for two of those years in Congress), Dennett moved away from the fray. Her decision to leave the political arena can be interpreted as a sign of retreat or an admission of outright defeat, but her vision continued to be publicized through her book *Birth Control Laws*. Dennett did not remain at the margins of the reform community for long. By 1929, she was facing charges for violating the Comstock Laws and using the U.S. Postal Service to mail obscene materials. Her subsequent trial repositioned her at the center of reform efforts to liberalize discussion and the flow of information about sexual matters. The trial also underscores the extent to which Dennett's formulation of the issues of pacifism, birth control, and sexual education were predicated on her dedication to individual liberties.

Obscenity, Publicity, and the Dennett Trial

In 1915 Dennett wrote an essay the purpose of which was to educate her teenage sons Carleton and Devon about sexual matters. Frustrated by available sex education texts, Dennett wrote frank descriptions of anatomy and sexual intercourse and included such topics as masturbation and orgasm. Attracting the attention of her friends, the little essay began to circulate and Dennett began to shop around for a publisher. Dennett's essay was published in 1918 in the *Medical Review of Reviews* as "The Sex Side of Life," reprinted in *The Modern School*, and then published in pamphlet form. The postmaster general banned it in 1922.

In *Who's Obscene?*, Dennett traced the history of her obscenity trial and argued that the ban was actually issued as a reprisal for her birth control activities. She wrote that there was "strong circumstantial evidence that the suppression was an act of retaliation due to official resentment of my work in another direction, rather than the contents of my pamphlet."[86] This claim likely reflected equal amounts of validity and paranoia, as earlier in the year

Dennett published an inflammatory article in the *BCH* that all but dared the postmaster general to try to enforce the Comstock Laws. She promptly received notice in the mail that "The Sex Side of Life" was unmailable under Section 211 of the penal code. Having made her reputation as a law-abiding reformer in contrast to the more controversial Sanger, Dennett uncharacteristically ignored this notice and continued to mail the pamphlet upon request. In January 1929 the U.S. Attorney's Office brought charges against Dennett for violating the federal Criminal Code. Her subsequent trial cemented her place in the civil liberties movement, and the ACLU came forward to defend her. Ironically, the publicity Dennett gained through her censorship trial brought her name into the limelight of the reform community that had virtually rejected her leadership and her agenda on birth control. The trial encouraged birth control reformers to rethink their strategies and loyalties; by the 1930s, many came around to supporting clean repeal over doctors-only legislation.[87] However, this change of heart would come too late to affect the course of the movement.[88]

Since the 1922 ban, Dennett had sent "Sex Side of Life" to interested parties—including educational, religious, and welfare organizations such as the YMCA and the Union Theological Seminary—via first-class mail. The postmaster general who brought legal action against Dennett claimed that his action was a response to a complaint by members of the Daughters of the American Revolution.[89] In April 1929, Dennett was convicted by the Federal District Court of Brooklyn for mailing indecent materials. Dennett faced a $300 fine, but no imprisonment, for her crime. She refused to pay any money on the same grounds on which she had based her political career, that is, freedom of speech and information. In a letter to her supporters, she wrote, "If the Government wishes to penalize me for my educational work, it must stand the shame of making it a prison sentence. The Government is disgraced, not I."[90]

During her trial, Dennett discovered she had some unlikely supporters and suffered the loss of supposed allies. For example, despite its growing problems with Sanger (which will be chronicled in the next chapter), the Birth Control League of Massachusetts (BCLM) refused to pass a resolution of protest on her behalf. Dr. Antoinette Konikow, a member of the BCLM who had earlier been a victim of obscenity laws, apologetically explained to Dennett that "our Executive Committee is now dealing with the 'nicest' physicians in Boston and probably will be afraid to take a stand."[91]

After Dennett's conviction, Konikow wrote again that, "The Birth Control League here is under Professor East's influence and he is . . . always afraid. The only energetic person in the crowd is Mrs. Oakes

[Blanche] Ames."[92] Despite Konikow's criticism, however, the executive secretary of the BCLM did send Dennett a letter of condolence upon her conviction, writing, "The BCLM sends you its deepest sympathy for your trial and the unfair way in which it was handled and the hope that you will be given another and just trial."[93] The ABCL's *BCR* also expressed sympathy and a bit more outrage when it published the following satirical account of the Dennett trial: "Denied expert testimony, twelve men carefully selected for their advanced years and comparative ignorance took it upon themselves to decide a question demanding wide knowledge and modern minds. . . . If we no longer use the rack and screws, we still have jails for those who dare to speak out."[94]

Dennett's indictment inspired the ACLU to set up a defense committee; a great deal of protest was aroused among liberal circles. Among those who testified at her trial or sent letters of support were John Dewey, Dr. Robert Dickinson, Rabbi Stephen Wise, H. L. Mencken, and Katherine Bemont Davis. In her account of the trial, Dennett remembered that "public protest against any verdict of guilty was instantaneous."[95] Foremost among her supporters was the ACLU, which supplied her defense counsel for the trial, raised money, and provided publicity.[96] Established in 1917, the ACLU focused primarily on labor and political speech in its first decade. A few lawyers in the organization sought to expand into other arenas of free speech. Morris Ernst, for example, published *To the Pure* in 1928 in which he bitterly attacked existing obscenity statutes. Ernst actively sought cases with which he might test the constitutionality of the Comstock Laws and offered his services free of charge to Dennett and, later, to Margaret Sanger. The Dennett case has been credited with facilitating the expansion of the ACLU agenda to include all forms of censorship and to overcome its reticence to litigate cases with an overt sexual content.[97] Although the Dennett trial moved the ACLU into uncharted territory, it served to reinforce Dennett's already established commitment to civil liberties: "The day is surely coming when American citizens and their Congressmen will realize that the laws which give to Post Office officials the power to penalize anyone they see fit to select as their victim, are totally at variance with justice and wisdom, and the principles on which our government was founded."[98]

In March 1930, Judge Augustus Hand of the Federal Court of Appeals reversed the district court's guilty verdict, setting an important precedent in obscenity law. He repudiated the precedent upon which earlier obscenity cases were tried: they labeled as obscene any material that might stimulate prurient interest in any individual. Hand argued that, although works dealing with sexual matters might arouse passions, this could not be an accurate test of obscenity. In writing his decision to reverse the conviction, he took Dennett's intent into account. The precedent set in the Dennett trial alleviated a major legal barrier to sex education in the United States.[99]

On the heels of her highly publicized victory, Dennett expanded her rationale for an open birth control bill to include touting its advantages in the arena of sex education. Despite her failures as a lobbyist and strategist for the birth control movement, Dennett's obscenity indictment bolstered her earlier conviction that birth control should be fought for on an anticensorship platform. She now argued that, "the primary need for the clean repeal is not so much that it will facilitate the circulation of contraceptive knowledge, as that it will help to clean up the public mind. It is a great stroke in sex education, and as such is invaluable at this stage of the birth control movement."[100] Thus, in the wake of her trial, Dennett moved even farther away from the question of provision and toward free speech and education. This move further facilitated her alienation from the reproductive reform mainstream, as the CB tried desperately to protect and expand provision of services to mothers and children, and Sanger continued to work tirelessly to open clinics.[101]

Dennett took full advantage of her publicity to position herself at the center of a progressive movement that celebrated freedom of speech and included issues of sexuality in the realm of legitimate, protected discourse. She expressed optimism that "this absurd mess may be helpful in precipitating more rapid progress toward the abolition of Post Office censorship and the renovation of the laws in regard to birth control. . . . [T]he prosecution is really an aftermath of my work on the Federal bill, so although the little pamphlet had nothing to do with birth control, the prosecution has."[102]

During her trial, Dennett rarely missed an opportunity to refer back to her earlier work in the birth control movement. Her legal troubles brought her publicity on a par with Sanger's earlier moments in the public eye. This exposure coincided with growing problems between Sanger and her former colleagues in the ABCL, which Dennett also made sure to capitalize on. By the fall of 1929, Dennett received a letter from the executive secretary of the ABCL confirming her participation in the next International Birth Control Conference. This invitation represented a clear shift from the earlier days, when Sanger's leadership of the ABCL ensured Dennett's silence at conferences. Since those days, the ABCL had made the most of Sanger's distraction with her federal and clinical projects to gather courage to defy her. This letter revealed the organization's evolving political agenda and the fault lines that had begun to shake the foundations of Sanger's uncontested leadership.

No one will be better able than you to handle the arguments for the dele-tion of the words 'prevention of conception' from the federal obscenity laws. Many of our Board have become converted to that point of view. The only reason that I have ever been for a limited bill was that it might be more pos-sible to pass one than to get a bill wiping all restrictions off the statute books through Congress.[103]

Dennett was rejuvenated by this trend and delighted to describe the dis-sension in Sanger's ranks to her friends and colleagues. She interpreted the problem between the ABCL and Sanger as a consequence of Sanger's faulty diplomacy and political strategy. Sanger left the League specifically to work on federal legislation without inviting any ABCL officials to join her new group. Once opinions other than Sanger's official one began to trickle out of the ABCL, Dennett reaped the benefits of the new open-ness. Even the president of the ABCL, Eleanor Jones, invited Dennett to speak at a luncheon discussion on the topic of federal legislation in the fall of 1929.[104]

The result of Dennett's friendly association with the ABCL convinced her that the tide was finally turning in a more hospitable direction. After spending time with the president and the executive secretary of the ABCL, Dennett confirmed her suspicion that both women now opposed Sanger's doctors-only bill, but were unwilling to take a public stand against her. Both women relayed stories of Sanger's tyrannical and irre-sponsible behavior; Dennett interpreted their candidness and friendliness as evidence of their imminent defection from the Sanger camp. Ten years after her unsuccessful attempts to pass an open bill, Dennett saw the mainstream rank-and-file reformers moving closer to her and further away from Sanger. Utterly gratified and optimistic, Dennett told VPL president Myra Gallert that, if after her speech before the ABCL in November the ABCL decided in favor of an open bill, it seemed logical for the two organizations to merge, that is, for the VPL to join the ABCL. By February 1930, Dennett stated with conviction that she had no doubt that the ABCL would officially and publicly come out in favor of an open bill within the year.[105] However, even by the end of 1930 Jones refrained from public defection.

I was much pleased that you and Mrs. Gallert should invite me to serve on the VPL National Council, and I should have been glad to do so, to show my sympathy with the aims of the League. But I felt that before accepting I ought to consult the other directors of the ABCL, and they, I am sorry to say, feel that in view of the ABCL's endorsement of the "doctors-only bill,"

it would be unadvisable for the president to make public her personal
endorsement of the "open bill," even though . . . two of our directors have
already done so.[106]

Jones sounded genuinely disappointed that she was unable to make
public her political preference for the open bill, and Dennett responded
sympathetically.

The private conversions of certain prominent members of the ABCL
spurred Dennett's convictions as to the righteousness of her agenda.
Indeed, Dennett's trial had supplied her with a broad group of supporters,
much needed publicity, and a new level of confidence. She exploited her
experience of governmental censorship to emphasize the fundamental
need for free speech in a democratic society. In fact, by 1931, Dennett's
was emboldened to confront Sanger. Dennett cautioned Sanger not to let
their personal relationship factor into her political decisions, but to objec-
tively acknowledge "the absurdity of a limited bill" when the movement
has already come so far.[107]

Dennett's arguments served to convert not just important ABCL
board members, but rank-and-file birth control supporters. A woman
from California even took it upon herself to write to Sanger to ask that
she change her tactics. Her letter illuminates the key difference between
Dennett's clean repeal and Sanger's doctors-only strategy.

> Let us have a clean status for birth control. It must be free to everyone, just
> for the asking, without any strings thereto. . . . Why is the Government so
> concerned over births only to wipe out lives by the wholesale when they are
> old enough to be of some use in the world. Here is hoping that mothers of
> men will have everything to say about their own children, and men and
> Government nothing. You are the one to fix it right.[108]

This letter highlights a frustrating situation for Dennett: she had origi-
nated a rationale for birth control that had become the more popular one
by the early 1930s, but could not compete with Sanger in the realm of
leadership and renown. Thus, even energy devoted to clean repeal was
sometimes directed toward Sanger as she, and not Dennett, seemed the
"one to fix it right."

ᘓᛇᘔ

Although the economic depression of the 1930s brought enormous suffering for many Americans, it actually served the birth control movement

well. Economic hardship and a new commitment on the part of the federal government to respond to those in need made it easier than ever before to convince politicians of the need for family limitation. As more families needed public relief and as family size directly impacted economic status, the demand for birth control became linked with other plans for economic recovery (at least in the public mind, if not in public policy). Sanger and the ABCL, which had always used economic arguments as part of its campaign, found in the economic depression a great opportunity to plead their case. Dennett, however, shied away from economic arguments just when they seemed to be working most effectively, instead continuing to make an appeal for civil liberties. Whether principled or merely obstinate, Dennett's choices in the 1930s mirrored her decision in the 1920s to reject medicalization despite its promised political advantages.

Dennett's problems with the ACLU in this period highlight her staunch commitment to justice in the face of a movement turning increasingly to pragmatic economic rationales for reform. Although the ACLU had provided counsel and support for Dennett during her trial in 1929, she perceived the organization's commitment to birth control as shallow and unreliable. On December 8, 1934, she sent a telegram to Roger Baldwin, president of the ACLU, warning him not to come out in support of Sanger's doctors-only bill at the ACLU conference in Washington, D.C. Baldwin wrote an ambiguous response to her appeal:

> We wrestled with this very question last year and our Board of Directors came to the conclusion that we could not endorse exclusively a bill to make birth control legal in the mails only when endorsed by medical agencies. We did endorse the limited bill as a step toward the complete abolition of all control over birth control information, realizing that practically it constitutes an issue which has a chance of favorable consideration. We have always made it clear that this is not the goal we are seeking.[109]

Dennett had little patience with Baldwin's explanation of how the ACLU could at once support both Sanger's and her own legislative strategies, as they seemed to her to be utterly incompatible. She argued that Baldwin was "an incorrigible wobbler on this birth control legislative question," but that she still expected him "to stay put some fine day."[110] While Baldwin could argue that Sanger's bill was a natural precursor to Dennett's goal of clean repeal, Dennett regarded this position as ideologically timid and unsound. Either the ACLU would unconditionally and vocally support civil liberties, or it would betray its most basic tenets.

Endorsing a limited permissive exemption bill is a queer business for the
Civil Liberties Union, isn't it? Establishing special privilege is hardly a step
toward freedom or equality, is it? Legalizing class monopoly is not quite in
line with the Union's general principles, is it? . . . Even if it were easier to
pass a limited bill than a repeal bill, which isn't so, is it worth while to do
it, at the expense of one's principles regarding special privilege and civil
liberties?[111]

Baldwin replied that he and his organization were in basic agreement with
Dennett but that modification of a bad law was better than no progress at
all. He challenged her assessment of the ACLU's support of a doctors-bill
as a compromise of its principles, asserting that this endorsement was
merely a practical step to take.[112]

Dennett had to contend with others in the ranks who chose practical
steps over what she considered principled integrity. Even as her relations
with high-ranking officials in the ABCL became more cordial, and their
views more compatible, Dennett felt frustrated with what she perceived
as her singular dedication to long-term considerations and principles of
justice. In her book, *Who's Obscene?*, she would lament that, "the compromise that is so often made with the hypothetical unreadiness of others to
move ahead forms one of the most disheartening factors in social
progress."[113]

In 1936 Marguerite Benson of the ABCL asked Dennett for her
advice regarding the League's strategy. Benson contended that legislative
reform took too much time and energy away from the immediate goal of
providing birth control information and materials to the greatest number
of women. She also argued that an enlightened public considered prohib-
itive birth control laws archaic, as evidenced by the numerous birth control clinics now "operating in the light of day."[114] Although Dennett
assured Benson that she would "feel as you do about soft pedaling the
legality question—just for the sake of speeding up the establishment of
clinics and lessening the timidity of doctors," she reminded her that, "the
situation with regard to birth control laws seems to involve two rather separate considerations, the short run and the long run accomplishments."
Dennett argued that both were "important for public welfare."[115] She
agreed that, in the short run, getting information and materials to as many
people as possible was of vital importance. In that regard, Dennett con-
curred that "court interpretations rather than amendments or repeal acts,
are of great aid to the program." However, Dennett warned that the birth
control movement should not abandon its principles in favor of expediency.

The long-run consideration is to have laws which say what they mean and mean what they say, the sort which can be respected by the public and enforced by the government. This is a civic and educational consideration, rather than one of health in the immediate sense. Whittling away the meaning of the present laws by a succession of loop-hole decisions is an immensely clever use of legal talent. . . . Yet, while these decisions do instant good . . . they do not take the place of definite law revision, and they are actually detrimental on two counts. First, they use a method which anti-social interests can and do use successfully. . . . Second, these decisions make a monkey of the law, and contribute yet another bit to undermining respect and lessening confidence in the integrity of the law in general.[116]

Thus, Dennett made it clear to Benson that she had some sympathy with the tactic of relying on judicial interpretation rather than aggressively seeking legislative change, but that this strategy also had its flaws. She argued that she saw herself as both a reformer and a citizen and that the latter affiliation forced her to consider larger questions with regard to birth control laws. Dennett ended her letter on a cordial note, stressing that "we are doubtless both headed for the same ultimate goal."[117]

Although making progress in converting mainstream birth control reformers to Dennett's perspective in the wake of her trials, her campaign faltered in the face of the *U.S. v. One Package* court decision. In 1936 Judge Hand of the Second Circuit Court ruled in that case that the Comstock Law should be interpreted as covering "only such articles as Congress would have denounced as immoral if it had understood all the conditions under which they were to be used."[118] He went on to argue that the purpose of the Comstock Law "was not to prevent the importation, sale, or carriage by mail of things which might intelligently be employed by conscientious and competent physicians for the purpose of saving life or promoting the well-being of their patients."[119] Thus, in giving unrestricted authority to physicians, the *One Package* decision promoted Sanger's strategies rather than Dennett's. While Sanger and supporters of the doctors-only strategy could hail the *One Package* decision as "the greatest legal victory in the birth control movement," Dennett was not satisfied in the least with this ruling.[120] She regarded *One Package* as she did the doctors-only strategy as a whole: as a compromised position and one that would ultimately be regretted.[121]

Sanger spent the months after the court decision spreading information to physicians and public health officers. By early 1937, she decided to dissolve the National Committee on Federal Legislation for Birth

Control. This decision ultimately led the way for the formation of the Planned Parenthood Federation of America. Her domestic agenda realized, Sanger moved onto the international scene in the 1940s and 1950s, securing her reputation as the undisputed worldwide leader of the birth control movement.

Dennett found it difficult to convince fellow birth control advocates that more needed to be done after the *One Package* ruling. Her obscenity trial lawyer, Morris Ernst, for example, argued that the ruling represented "the last word on the subject," predicting that state courts would surely follow the federal precedent.[122] In the face of such an atmosphere of confidence, Dennett's warnings went largely unheeded. Although both Dennett and Sanger had been proven wrong in their decision to attempt legislative reform, which continued to offer no relief, the *One Package* decision did seem to validate Sanger's rationale behind the doctors-only strategy; it did not alter social mores around the use of birth control, but clarified the right of physicians to offer a fuller range of reproductive health services to their patients. But the *One Package* decision did not protect birth control clinics that employed nurses or social workers; nor did it protect women who sought birth control for "merely personal" reasons. The flaws inherent in the choice to rely on this decision will be made clear in the next chapter, which traces the history of the birth control movement in Massachusetts throughout the 1930s.

After 1936, Dennett's political activism slowed down, as she once again took up her work as an artisan. She even attempted to obtain a government commission for her art work during the depression, arguing that "it would seem to be at least poetic, if no other sort of justice, for the Government to make up, somewhat, for the very damaging blunder of its Post Office official."[123] Dennett never received a commission for her work, and her leather work failed to bring her much income or fame. During the last decade of her life, she continued her membership in various clubs and organizations, including the VPL, Heterodoxy, the Women's Peace Union, and the Society of Arts and Crafts.

Dennett's death in a nursing home in Valatie, New York, in 1947 meant that, unlike Sanger, she would not live to see birth control become a constitutionally protected right of married couples in the Supreme Court decision *Griswold v. Connecticut*. This 1965 ruling would have pleased Dennett to the extent that it reflected her commitment to individual rights and freedom from government interference. However, as history has shown in the cases of both birth control and abortion, constitutional protection can mean something quite different than does the actual provision of health care services. In this sense, the historical record has illuminated the flaws in the strategies of both Sanger and Dennett. While the former led a movement that prioritized the rights of physicians and concerns about population over women's individual rights, the latter kept the concept of individual rights at the center of her vision while neglecting the extent to which the lives of real people would be improved by those rights. In other words, Dennett's notion of justice was predicated on a sense of democracy, but not equality. She believed that the government should allow people to make their own decisions regarding the most intimate aspects of their reproductive and sexual lives, but never questioned how this decision-making power might be undermined by such factors as poverty or ignorance. Sanger, on the other hand, like the majority of female reformers struggling for women's reproductive health and rights, directly addressed the question of provision. Her interest in making sure that women got the birth control information and devices they needed led her in unintended directions; namely, into a battle for the rights of physicians and the adoption of eugenics rhetoric that ultimately threatened women's reproductive autonomy.

Unlike the most well-known female reformers in the Progressive Era and interwar years, Dennett buttressed a commitment to reproductive reform with skepticism about state activism and a conscious decision to eschew maternalist politics. She framed the birth control struggle as a fight for liberty, rather than a push for social welfare, and therefore focused on questions of access rather than on demands for the provision of goods and services. Thus, her orientation diverged from state-sponsored solutions and strategies to aid women. As was the case with Dummer, Dennett's work on birth control would lead her to confront and challenge sexual mores: Dummer, because they oppressed women and children, and Dennett, because they kept all people ignorant through the censorship that she abhorred.

4

"To do a real amount of good
. . . without raising antagonism"

BLANCHE AMES, LOCAL CIRCUMSTANCES,
AND BIRTH CONTROL POLITICS

Like Mary Dennett, Blanche Ames (1878–1961) dedicated her life to social reform, first in the suffrage movement and then, for the next twenty years, as a leader of the birth control movement. Ames kept aloof from both the VPL and the Sangerist wing of the birth control movement to construct her own statewide campaign in Massachusetts. Ames's relationship to Sanger was comparable to Dummer's with the women in the Children's Bureau; unlike Dennett, Ames did not consider herself a rival of, or harbor any personal animosity toward, Sanger. However, she did act as a constructive critic. Like Dennett, she provides an interesting foil for Sanger, as historians can compare the compromises each woman made and evaluate the efficacy and staying power of these choices.

Throughout the interwar years, Ames was simultaneously more cautious and more progressive than her cohorts in both Sanger's American Birth Control League (ABCL) and Dennett's Voluntary Parenthood League (VPL). On a personal level, she rejected a purely medical rationale for the use of birth control, yet actively sought the support of physicians in her own state in an effort to de-radicalize and popularize her cause. Ames displayed a progressive commitment to enlarging the scope of the birth control movement to include economic reasons for family limitation—especially once the economic depression of the 1930s brought unprecedented unemployment rates and widespread poverty—while at the same time attempting to gain support for her cause from conservative reformers in her own state, such as Elizabeth Lowell Putnam. These eclectic strategies make the story of the Massachusetts birth control movement important in terms of understanding the diverse tactics and

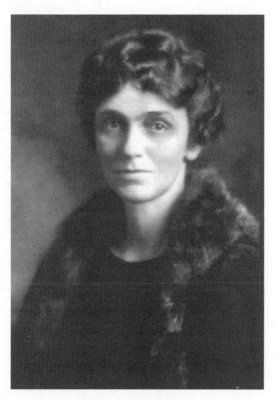

FIG. 4 BLANCHE AMES.
Photo courtesy of the Schlesinger Library, Radcliffe
Institute, Harvard University.

goals of reproductive reformers in the interwar years. Furthermore, Ames's choices muddied and defied categorization as she moved through various rhetorical and strategic stages. Therefore, her story illustrates not only the political diversity and creativity this study seeks to uncover, but also the varying degree of success that different political orientations yielded for reproductive reformers.

Ames was born in Lowell, Massachusetts, to a very well-entrenched and prominent New England family. Her father, General Adelbert Ames, served as governor of Mississippi during Reconstruction, and her maternal grandfather (Benjamin F. Butler) served as governor of Massachusetts. Her mother, Blanche Butler, supported women's suffrage and provided her daughter with a model of a civic-minded and independent woman.

Blanche spent most of her childhood in Lowell and then entered Smith College in 1895. In addition to their activist New England roots,

Ames and Dennett were both talented artists. At Smith, Blanche excelled in art, participated in athletics, and was elected president of her class. One year after graduating from Smith, Blanche married Oakes Ames, an instructor of botany at Harvard University and moved with him to North Easton, Massachusetts. The Ames's had four children.

Oakes and Blanche combined their expertise to create a seven-volume series on orchids, which Blanche illustrated. In addition to working as an illustrator, Blanche was active in civic affairs. Her first political passion was women's suffrage. As a young woman, Ames had lamented in her diary that, "Men always seem to have the advantage—in dress, in law, in politics—everything. Will the time ever come when it will be equally easy for women to exist?"[1] In 1913, two years before the state legislature passed and submitted to voters a constitutional amendment granting women suffrage, Ames set out to even the score through suffrage work. In this year, she joined the Ways and Means Committee of the Massachusetts Woman Suffrage Association (MWSA). This move launched her impressively active career in the state suffrage movement, which involved her chairing suffrage festivals, organizing open-air rallies, serving as president of her town suffrage league and treasurer of the MWSA, and utilizing her artistic talents to create a series of popular pro-suffrage political cartoons.[2]

As in Dennett's case, Ames's experiences in the suffrage movement shaped her political perspective. As a leader of the Massachusetts suffrage movement, Ames had first-hand knowledge of the power of conservative forces in her home state. Massachusetts boasted the first organization opposed to women's suffrage in the country. Due at least in part to its influence, Ames and her pro-suffrage allies and suffered a devastating defeat in the state suffrage referendum of 1915. In contrast to their colleagues in New York, whose defeat spurred them to new levels of energy, the Massachusetts suffragists all but gave up their statewide campaign after 1915. Ames surely knew that the well-organized antisuffrage forces, made up of conservative politicians and their constituents and a large bloc of Catholic voters, would also spell trouble for the fledgling birth control movement. In this context, the frustrations and peculiar predilections that shaped her birth control work make more sense.

Even before the Nineteenth Amendment had passed, Ames turned her attention to the other feminist cause that would shape her life's work: birth control. She co-founded the Birth Control League of Massachusetts (BCLM) in 1916, and served as president of the League on and off until her resignation in 1935. Her activity on behalf of the legalization of birth control was marked by a cautious conservatism that was not always compatible with her personal commitments and beliefs. Her activities reflect the volatile and complex nature of reproductive rights politics in the early twentieth century. Although Ames believed in self-determination and equality for women, the struggle for birth control that she led in Massachusetts for two decades was marked by deference to medical authority and political timidity. Her career illustrates how one's personal views on motherhood and womanhood cannot necessarily be equated with the political strategies and tactics one ultimately utilizes. A resolute feminist, Ames became an expert at compromise who molded her reform campaign to fit her locale.

This chapter will examine Ames's political career in the birth control movement, focusing on the evolution of her ideas and her strategy to make state-level reform a priority over federal reform. Massachusetts holds a unique place in the history of reproductive reform. One of only three states to reject the Sheppard-Towner Act and one of the last states to legalize birth control, Massachusetts provides historians with a clear picture of the political obstacles facing reproductive rights and reproductive health reformers. Citizen activists from prominent families could be found across the political spectrum. Putnam exemplified the elite Brahmin conservatives who created a formidable antisuffrage movement, fought against federal "paternalism," and decried changing sexual mores. Ames, however, came from an activist family that was just as prominent and wealthy as Putnam's but boasted generations of liberal activists. Veterans of the Massachusetts suffrage fray, Ames and Dennett took decidedly different routes as they branched out into the birth control movement. Whereas Ames remained steadfast in her focus on state politics, Dennett instead chose to embark on a federal campaign. Both of these strategies resulted in alienation from Sanger and her wing of the movement. Both strategies also necessitated certain tactical maneuvers that have been lost in studies that concentrate on Sanger, but that help round out our understanding of the politics of reproductive reform.

Studying Ames and the BCLM remedies several historical myths: that Sanger was virtually omnipotent in shaping the contours of the American birth control movement (and that understanding the national organizations will provide an adequate portrait of the movement), that the birth control movement was quite distant from related reproductive health reform issues, and that both the medicalization strategy and reliance on judicial review were politically successful. Whereas the previous chapter highlighted the relative success of Sanger's doctors-only strategy over Dennett's efforts at clean repeal of the Comstock Laws, this chapter will further contextualize and complicate assessment of the movement. Ames's career reveals other major fault lines within the birth control movement:

debates over the necessity or efficacy of legislative reform to advance the cause, coalition-building strategies, and—as we have seen with Dennett's career—the level of commitment to individual rights.

⟨⟩

In 1916 a group of prominent Boston citizens formed the Allison Defense Committee in response to the indictment of Van Kleek Allison, a layperson arrested for distributing birth control literature to working women in the North End of Boston. This group soon changed its name to the Birth Control League of Massachusetts (BCLM), and elected Blanche Ames as its president.

The BCLM sought to educate Massachusetts citizens about contraception and work for its legalization. It succeeded in, and maintained a commitment to, the former task to a much greater degree than it did to the latter. The League attracted publicity through public meetings and outreach to state women's clubs as a result of the conscious effort of activists to follow through on high hopes that birth control would become part of the mainstream female reform agenda. As one of its first projects, the BCLM decided to explore the scope of prohibitions in the state penal code to clear up any confusion about the legality of contraceptive advice, distribution, and use.

Despite the overarching force of the federal Comstock Laws, which categorized birth control information and devices as obscenities to be prohibited by the post office, state statutes varied in degree and intent. Most statutes repressed the flow of information about birth control to some degree. Many states had prohibitions against publishing, advertising, or distributing information on contraception. Colorado specifically forbade the transportation of contraceptives into the state, and Connecticut had a state law that prohibited the use of birth control.[3] In the context of such variation, it was not unusual for state leagues to begin their work on the birth control issue by seeking clarification of the law.[4] This process, however, did not always yield concrete or satisfying answers. This was certainly the case in Massachusetts.

On the basis of legal opinions from prominent lawyers, the League learned that, despite severe prohibitions in Massachusetts, loopholes did exist through which the BCLM might operate. Massachusetts law prohibited the distribution of printed materials related to contraception and the manufacture of any drug or instrument for contraception. However, the League's lawyer advised its members that there existed no reference in the state penal code to oral information about contraception or any prohibition against the maintenance of an office where such information could be provided. For league members, this loophole provided some hope that practical work could be accomplished. Soon, however, another lawyer advised the BCLM to proceed with caution. He argued that state statutes contained hidden dangers: "It is true that our statutes have reference to *printed* and not to *oral* communication, so that doctors, nurses, and individuals may . . . give oral information. The statute does not prohibit the maintenance of an office where such information may be given, *but no printed matter can be circulated giving any "hint" that such information can be had there. Even the name of the League itself on the door or on cards or on letterhead may be deemed to give such a "hint" and therefore be prohibited."*[5] This somewhat alarmist opinion was written in 1917 by Prescott Hall, a founding member of the BCLM's executive committee. His words both shaped and mirrored the overwhelming cautiousness that characterized the organization. The League had attracted citizens who were prominent and progressive, but not necessarily interested in breaking the law. In this respect, most members of the BCLM were more akin to Dennett than Sanger in this period: not comfortable with radical tactics, but determined to work for the cause. As we have seen, in 1917 two major models existed for local birth control reformers to follow or reject: Sanger's radical calls for civil disobedience published in both the *Woman Rebel* and the *BCR* and exemplified by her arrest for opening an illegal clinic, and Dennett and the National Birth Control League's commitment to reforming laws in an "orderly and proper manner." The BCLM rejected both models as too activist, opting instead to avoid overt confrontation with the law and accommodate itself to the peculiarities of the Massachusetts penal code.

A successful strategy for operating in a way consistent with Massachusetts laws did not evolve for two years. In the interim, the Massachusetts Supreme Court convicted Allison, and the United States entered World War I. The BCLM did not emerge intact from these setbacks. Birth control activists in Massachusetts had to reconceptualize their cause to fit the postwar world and the realities of state laws. Within this context, the birth control movement in Massachusetts, led by an ardent yet pragmatic Blanche Ames, moved in some surprising directions.

In 1919, the same year that Dennett launched her federal lobbying campaign, the advisory board of the BCLM decided to change the name of the organization to the Family Welfare Foundation (FWF). Ames described this shift in a letter to the members of the BCLM, explaining, "During the war it was considered inadvisable to push the work of the League and now, instead of going ahead again along the old lines, it seems more expedient to organize a new league with a broader, more constructive policy."[6] Expediency certainly characterized the new FWF. It sought to avoid all controversy and to associate itself with the most respectable causes and classes of people. Not only was the term "birth control" absent from the new name, but these words also never appeared in any literature put out by the FWF. At times, significant creative efforts were taken to soft-pedal the objectives of the Foundation. For example, in one attempt to describe its new function, the FWF claimed that it would "acquire and disseminate knowledge of value to individuals in all their family relationships, especially that of parenthood."[7] Birth controllers told themselves that the nominal change from the BCLM to the FWF was a legitimate response to the particular legal circumstances in Massachusetts. Looking back years later, though, Ames deemed the conservative climate after the war a primary instigator of this shift. Even at the time, Ames complained that the Foundation's objectives "were veiled and lacked human interest."[8] Despite her frustration with the Foundation, however, Ames remained president, and executed the conservative policies formulated by the board.

The broader, "more constructive," policies of the FWF certainly marked a contrast between what the FWF hoped to accomplish and both Sanger's and Dennett's activities. As seen in the previous chapter, whereas Sanger's early policy emphasized publicity, propaganda, and elements of civil disobedience to test the constitutionality and limits of birth control laws, Dennett worked to launch an unprecedented federal campaign to repeal the offending section of the Comstock Laws. Ames and other members of the BCLM discouraged these tactics in what they considered the more conservative state of Massachusetts.[9] The advisory board looked for ways in which the FWF might "do a real amount of good, both educational and practical, without raising antagonism."[10] As the board perceived it, raising antagonism did not merely refer to Sanger's radical rhetoric and tactics, but also included Dennett's lobbying efforts. The FWF's intention—"to do a real amount of good"—was both broad and vague, and its tactics reflected this. Under Ames's tutelage, the FWF dedicated itself to reducing risk and broadening appeal. Like Dennett's movement away from radical or confrontational tactics, Ames diverged from Sanger in adopting maternalist rhetoric. Less optimistic and perhaps less naïve about political circumstances, Ames sought to hitch her cause to a reliable wagon.

The change of name to the Family Welfare Foundation, however, was not merely a pragmatic response to legal restrictions and a conservative climate. It also represented a sincere attempt on the part of Boston reformers to broaden the scope of both their organization and the birth

control movement itself. Accordingly, after the war we see the first conscious efforts by reformers to associate birth control with more palatable
or popular reforms. Mainstream progressive reformers like Dennett and
Ames sought to rescue the cause from its marginal obscurity. Like Dennett, Ames attempted to move away from the radicalism associated with
sexual and moral implications of birth control. Ames thus designed a
campaign that stressed the conservation and quality of life, and the welfare of American families. Due largely to Julia Lathrop's Children's Year,
one of the few reform issues that successfully spanned the pre- and postwar periods was concern about infant mortality. Infant mortality both fos-
tered and reflected interest in maternal welfare and public health.

The newly formed FWF tried to capitalize on this concern by defining its aims as part of a larger eugenic, child-saving, profamily agenda. Dr.
Evangeline Young, a lecturer for the FWF, wrote to various women's clubs
in Massachusetts offering to lecture on one of the following subjects: The
Care of Mothers During Pregnancy, How to Have Healthy Babies, Conservation of Child and Maternal Life, Education for Parenthood, and
Eugenic Ideals for the American Family. It is unclear from this list
whether the subject of contraception would be broached in this series of
lectures. Indeed, the list reads as if it could have been a pamphlet series
created by the CB, rather than a birth control league.

The FWF was divided into three departments: child welfare, maternal
welfare, and general research and public education. The FWF's stated
aims were, "to co-operate with existing organizations, to exclude none of
the activities now under way but to include more: instead of emphasizing
one single branch or another, as has been done a little here, a little there,
in supplying pure milk, instructing mothers in pre- and postnatal care or
in organizing Little Mothers' Leagues, etc., to unify the whole, to make it
one broad movement including all and excluding none of the ways to
reduce the present waste of the lives of mothers and infants."[11] Also
included in this broad agenda was insurance for mothers at the time of
childbirth. Avoiding any mention of contraception, the FWF sought to
place birth control in what it deemed a larger, more appropriate context:
public health and eugenic campaigns that sought to lower mortality rates
of mothers and infants.[12] The Foundation presented an inclusive vision of
reproductive reform that seemed more in keeping with the maternal and
infant welfare agenda elaborated by the CB than Sanger's early calls for
women's freedom from bondage.

Evaluating this vision in the context of Dummer's work on reproductive reform provides an interesting picture of points of agreement and
divergence. Dummer and Ames both attempted to bring the issues of

reproductive rights and health together under one rubric, envisioning a holistic movement that supported both mothers and infants. However, Dummer's inclusion of *Mutterschutz* ideas meant that her notions of family welfare reflected a challenge to the cultural norms that placed mothers and children in precarious circumstances. Ames's FWF, like the CB, called for education and dissemination of information on parenting. Rather than challenging norms, Ames championed birth control information as part of the body of knowledge necessary to keep families fit. Like Dennett, Ames sought ways to draw attention away from birth control's radical potential to liberate women from the burdens of unwanted children. However, unlike Dennett, Ames emphasized how birth control might fit into a larger, more palatable social welfare agenda.

Birth control reformers, like many progressive reformers, hoped that the death and destruction of the war would be followed by a period of social rebirth. Attention to public health, frank discussion of sex and family life, and the final flowering of progressive hopes for government expansion had characterized the war years. Optimism flourished among reformers who felt assured that science and an expanded federal apparatus would conquer poverty, ill health, and unnecessarily high rates of infant and maternal mortality. The FWF appealed to people's sorrow over loss of life, trying, specifically, to associate the sacrifice of women's lives with those of soldiers in the public mind. Echoes of both Dummer and Putnam can be found in the Foundation's literature: "Medieval fatalism . . . still clouds the popular mind in matters surrounding the deaths of mothers in childbirth, and this feeling is largely due to the fact that while steps have been taken which have lowered the infant death rate considerably in the last decade, nothing whatever has been done to lower the maternal death rate. . . . We made much of our soldiers and well they deserve it; but now that the war is over and we are free from their care, let us take care of the mothers!"[13] The FWF attempted to associate birth control with social progress, racial advancement, and public health. However, in the course of this campaign, it failed on two accounts: first, it never gained the support of mainstream social welfare reformers of the CB, and, second, it squashed real birth control activism for almost an entire decade in Massachusetts.

As the FWF tried to reach out to a broader spectrum of the public, its members took pains to disassociate from Sanger. In an effort to soften their original aims by cloaking them in the rhetoric of maternal and infant welfare, members needed to remain distant from the controversy stirred up by Sanger and her colleagues through arrests, civil disobedience, and publicity stunts. Although one might assume that the FWF masked a more radical agenda because it feared legal ramifications, records show that the Foundation took its new, broadened, and sanitized agenda quite seriously. The Foundation's attempts to recruit conservative support for its new agenda reflected the genuineness of the FWF's watered-down aims. As we have seen, one such figure whom Massachusetts birth controllers sought to court with their revised program was antisuffragist and infant welfare reformer Elizabeth Lowell Putnam. In August 1919, Vera P. Lane, the general secretary of the FWF, wrote to Putnam to detail the changes that had been made in the organization since its initial contact with her in 1916. Lane referred to the Foundation's "broader more constructive policy" and called her attention to the new name.[14] Putnam never responded to the appeal by the FWF, but its attempt to associate with her makes clear the FWF's political orientation. Putnam was identified as a possible supporter because she had been president of the American Child Hygiene Association and, by the end of the war, had become quite wellknown in infant welfare circles due to her innovative experiment in prenatal care. That she vocally decried women's suffrage and had already expressed her disapproval of birth control seemed less important to the members of the FWF than her commitment to maternalism and her social position.

The FWF's decision to concentrate on amorphous educational work at the expense of political reform did not go unnoticed or unchallenged from outside state borders. Although Sanger had yet to embark on a federal reform agenda by this time, Dennett displayed concern about the transformation of the BCLM into the FWF.

In June 1919, Dennett wrote a letter imploring the FWF to support her political campaign to reform federal censorship laws. She wrote, "If, as you say, the birth control league is inactive, and your new organization . . . does not feel able to do anything but wish us well with our project for getting our measure passed by Congress, to whom *can* we look in Massachusetts for active help? . . . Do you not feel that your educational program can be more rapidly accomplished if you help to make rational parenthood more possible by helping to free contraceptive knowledge from the ban?"[15] The FWF, however, was unwilling to align itself with Dennett's activities. Ames wanted to remain free of federal political entanglements so as not to aggravate the situation in Massachusetts. Dennett was particularly frustrated with Ames's strategy. She wrote to an officer of the FWF in 1919 that she "had not heard a word from Mrs. Ames. I have written to her twice. I wish very much she would see the point of concentrating on Congress rather than exclusively on state work. If everybody would only join to get this federal law repealed, the state laws would all go down like a card house."[16] Dennett then criticized the FWF by frankly stating that, "I cannot help wishing that in the statement of your objects, you had made it a little clearer that Voluntary Parenthood is one of them."[17] Thus, even as Dennett was herself in the midst of avoiding controversy or confrontation in her federal campaign, she opposed the FWF's decision to virtually abandon its commitment to birth control. She must have also been surprised at the direction the Foundation had taken under Ames's leadership, for Ames had a reputation as an ardent and energetic reformer.[18]

FWF Secretary Vera P. Lane did remain in contact with Dennett during this conservative period and even ordered copies of her pro-birth control pamphlet, "Yes-But." Although Lane's letter to Putnam characterized the Foundation as leaning toward a conservative policy, she also assured Dennett in a letter that, "I am hoping that there will be some way by which these two organizations (referring to the VPL and the FWF) can cooperate. We are moving a little slowly just now, but hope soon to report progress."[19] Lane went so far as to ask Dennett for any suggestions for bolstering the organization. Only one month earlier, Lane had also written to Margaret Sanger to convey that she hoped to meet with her to discuss the plans of the FWF. Thus, in its effort to increase public support, the FWF succeeded in diluting its aims to the extent that, in 1919, it could simultaneously assure Dennett, Sanger, and Putnam—three reformers with very different political agendas—of its good intentions.

By the fall of 1919, the FWF had requested that its name be taken off the list of birth control organizations named in the *Birth Control Review*.[20] It also decided to make a "gift" of five thousand copies of Dennett's "Yes-But" to Sanger, relieved that she was "glad to take them off your hands."[21] The conservative political climate also encouraged resignations. For example, legal advisor Prescott Hall had complained to Ames in the spring of 1919 that the Foundation's lecturer Dr. Young was in the habit of breaking the postal laws with the literature she sent. He warned that the people on the advisory board shunned association with lawbreakers and would resign if Young could not be kept in line. By October, Hall resigned as vice president and chair of the executive committee. His defection to the ranks of the anti-immigration movement in order to keep out "those who most need birth control after they enter the country" reveals the challenges Ames faced in holding together a rather eclectic group of reformers. In February 1920, the FWF informed its members that it was terminating all activities. It would be eight years until birth control supporters in Massachusetts were once again contacted in an effort to regroup along yet another set of guidelines and strategies.

Years later, Ames would reflect on the virtual inactivity and stagnation of the Massachusetts birth control movement in these years immediately following the war, disassociating herself from the conservative trend. She said, "After the rejoicing over winning the vote . . . the members of the birth control league scattered. It was hard to arouse interest in birth control work; the treatment of radicals during the war and the attitude of officials under Mayor Curley's governorship made people cautious. Finally the conservatives prevailed and the League changed its name. . . . But its program roused little interest, contributions lagged, attendance at meetings was not enough to secure a quorum. The Foundation became inactive."[22] Ames's recollections reveal that she was personally frustrated with postwar trends, though she continued her leadership during this period. She faced external political repression and internal pressure toward conservatism. These two forces would continue to shape her career throughout the interwar years, forcing her to compromise and conciliate until she could no longer tolerate the politics of the League.

The FWF episode is significant for three reasons. First, it illustrates the relatively conservative orientation of many rank-and-file birth control activists when compared to the publicity stirred up by Sanger and the ambitious federal program launched by Dennett. Second, it highlights the desire of at least some birth controllers to identify themselves as maternalists, rather than feminists; that is, to view birth control as a means to shore up families and save the lives of mothers and babies rather than as a strategy to liberate women. Finally, the disappointing results of this episode point to yet another strategy gone awry. The fact that, by the 1920s, birth controllers had yet to design successful reform strategies contextualizes Sanger's and Dennett's various attempts to overcome political and cultural obstacles.

Birth control reformers in Massachusetts were not the only ones who experienced setbacks during the 1920s. The ABCL and its affiliates made unsuccessful attempts to change the state laws in New York, Connecticut, and Pennsylvania during this decade. Sanger's biographer has asserted that on a national level, the movement "advanced only tentatively through the 1920s."[23] Among other things, this decade witnessed the failure of Dennett's and Sanger's federal reform campaigns; Sanger's resignation from the ABCL; the rejection of birth control as an issue by both the League of Women Voters and the National Women's Party; and several instances of police raids, arrests, and censorship.[24] One major lesson birth controllers learned during this frustrating decade was the importance of coalition building. The 1920s marked a period of stagnation for a movement that reached out to social welfare reformers, social workers, feminists, and maternalists. All of its advances rejected, the movement would soon turn to another group—medical professionals—that inspired it to reinvent itself once again.

Throughout the 1920s, Ames continued her political activities to a minor degree while focusing her energy on botanical illustration, which was the other major interest in her adult life. During these years, while on hiatus from the birth control movement, Ames worked with her husband to finish their major work in the field of economic botany, "Ames Charts of Economic Plants." Ames continued to receive correspondence during the 1920s from the American Birth Control League, the Massachusetts League of Women Voters, The Women's Committee for World Disarmament, the International Women's Suffrage Alliance, the Bryn Mawr Summer School for Women Working in Industry, and the Young Women's Christian Association. As was the case for many female reformers in the postwar, postsuffrage period, Ames's political life faltered and atomized in the 1920s just as she achieved a great deal of personal success in her field as an illustrator. According to Joan Jensen and Lois Scharf's examination of the women's movement in the interwar years, this pattern was a common one for accomplished women in this era.[25]

The BCLM Reincarnated: Courting Doctors

The next burst of birth control activity in Massachusetts was inspired by the arrest of Dr. Antoinette Konikow in February 1928 for giving a lecture on "sex hygiene." Specifically, Konikow was charged with exhibiting contraceptive devices. A revolutionary socialist, purported abortionist, and contributor to radical periodicals, Konikow had questionable associations that could have easily led members of the defunct FWF to disregarded her problems with the law. However, despite Konikow's radical orientation and affiliations, above all she was a physician. This fact would make all the difference to her potential supporters in Massachusetts. Although Konikow was acquitted one month after her arrest, birth control supporters formed a defense fund that ultimately turned into the second incarnation of the Birth Control League of Massachusetts, with Blanche Ames again acting as president. That this latest victim of the Massachusetts penal code was a physician fit nicely with the emerging medical orientation of the birth control movement. Dr. Konikow's arrest allowed the BCLM to resurrect itself as the champion of a new movement for physicians' rights, thereby perpetuating its tendency to avoid the feminist implications of birth control.

By 1928 the national movement for the legalization of birth control had undergone many changes since Margaret Sanger burst onto the scene in 1914 with her first issue of the *Woman Rebel*. One year after the FWF folded, the controversy between Sanger and Dennett erupted with the resignation of Dennett from the board of directors of the *Birth Control Review*. This move was inspired by Sanger's decision to begin a campaign for legislation that would ensure the legality of contraceptive advice and use only under the supervision of a physician. As the previous chapter has shown, this controversy heated up in 1924 when Sanger began working toward the passage of a federal law that would exempt doctors from the laws prohibiting the dissemination of birth control–related information and materials. Her decision was partially based on the fact that, throughout the 1920s, attempts at state reform were still largely unsuccessful. Sanger reasoned, like Dennett had earlier, that setting a precedent on the federal level would speed the reform process. By the mid-1920s, Sanger decided that public opinion had been significantly enlightened about the issue of birth control and that physicians could be persuaded to join in an effort that ensured their monopoly over the dissemination of contraceptives.

One month after Dr. Konikow's arrest in Massachusetts in 1928, Sanger resigned as president of the ABCL to devote her full attention to transforming the federal law along these lines. By 1929, she formed and led the National Committee of Federal Legislation for Birth Control. Sanger's clout ensured that most state leagues would acclimate to this new strategy, which emphasized federal legislation and a solely medical rationale for the use of birth control. In Massachusetts, however, reformers would reject the former and support the latter, thereby choosing Sanger over Dennett in support for doctors-only legislation but rejecting both women's attempts at prioritizing federal reform.

Sanger's strained relationship with the medical community in the 1920s and 1930s has been well documented by other historians.[26] Although never willing to give up control over the movement to physicians, once she began fighting for doctors-only legislation, she acknowledged that she needed the support and the clout of the medical profession. In 1929, police raided Sanger's Maternity Research Council, a New York clinic attempting both to provide contraceptive services to women under the legal exception recognized by Judge Crane in Section 1145 of the New York penal code, and to conduct a study of birth control practices and their safety and efficacy. Two doctors and two nurses were arrested, and case records of 150 patients were confiscated. This incident motivated the medical profession—at least in New York—to protest against misuse of the state police power and infringement upon the confidentiality of the physician-patient relationship. What followed was a power struggle between Sanger and New York doctors to control the direction of the movement that saw Sanger simultaneously fighting for doctors-only legislation and remaining committed to a birth control movement that endorsed eugenic, social, economic, and personal rationales for its use. In Massachusetts, on the other hand, birth controllers actively sought the alliance of doctors and then subordinated themselves to their wishes.

One month after the BCLM was reestablished, Ames wrote to the VPL asking for a copy of Dennett's book, *Birth Control Laws*. The new organization had decided to tackle legislative reform, at least on the state level, and needed Dennett's work to eliminate any misconceptions about the restrictions it faced. Indeed, the BCLM would spend most of its time in the first two to three years of its revitalization collecting information and legal opinions on Massachusetts' birth control statutes. The continuities, which ran through the first BCLM, the FWF, and now the second incarnation of the BCLM, lay in cautiousness over law breaking and commitment to tackling state rather than federal reform.

The new BCLM differed from past efforts in two significant ways: first, in defining birth control as a physician's issue rather than a maternalist one, and, second, in deciding to reform rather than accommodate itself to state laws. These changes were based on three important factors: the particularities of the Massachusetts legal code, the gradual decrease in the level of opposition to birth control among the medical community at large, and Sanger's move in these directions (medicalization and legislative reform). Birth control activists in Massachusetts were cautious but savvy political actors who responded to their environment and acknowledged the ebb and flow of political fortunes. Whereas in the years immediately following World War I the FWF sought to gain approval by associating itself with the more "respectable" causes of infant and maternal welfare and eugenics, by the late 1920s the Children's Bureau had faced the devastating loss of Sheppard-Towner as well as efforts to cut its funding, remove it from the Department of Labor, and collapse it into the U.S. Public Health Service. The power and respectability that birth controllers sought through alliances seemed now to lay with the organized medical community. According to one historian, "Nothing could bring greater prestige to contraception than to have it associated with the triumphant magic of medical science."[27]

Despite Ames's decision to proceed along the same lines as Sanger did (that is, working to secure physicians' right to prescribe birth control to their patients), she remained unwilling to reach beyond state borders. For this reason, the BCLM announced that it would sever its official association with the ABCL "until methods of approach become more nearly identical."[28] In an account of the three organizations working for birth control in Massachusetts, Ames made sure to distinguish between the ABCL, the BCLM, and Sanger's National Committee on Federal Legislation. She argued that each organization was independent and had a different scope, overlapping with the others only in terms of membership. While the ABCL was a national organization and the National Committee worked on federal legislation, Ames claimed that her own organization was, "absorbed with problems peculiar to Massachusetts; its methods of work are those suited to conservative Massachusetts people."[29] Thus, Ames resolved to accommodate her movement to the particularities of the political climate.

Massachusetts birth control reformers faced political challenges beyond those posed by the strict legal code prohibiting access to birth control information and materials. Throughout the 1910s and 1920s, an unlikely coalition of old-stock Republicans and Catholic conservatives rejected a number of significant progressive initiatives, including Sheppard-Towner, education reform and consolidation, and the Child Labor Amendment. According to Massachusetts historian Joseph Huthmacher, "In their opposition to centralization and control, newer American Catholics found themselves aligned with economic conservatives who also deprecated expansion of government power."[30] Thus, Roman Catholics echoed people like Putnam and her friends in the state house in railing against federal maternity aid and compulsory physical education programs; they feared that these programs would open the door to sex hygiene instruction and birth control propaganda for both children attending public schools and their mothers.[31] In this difficult climate, Ames's decision to concentrate on the peculiarities of Massachusetts politics, thereby distancing her group from the federal campaign, makes tactical sense.

According to legal opinions delivered after the revitalization of the League, the state penal code—while not providing a simple exemption for physicians (as found in New York's Section 1145)—lent itself to an interpretation that *could* exempt physicians from prohibitions regarding birth control. One of the BCLM's new legal advisors, C. R. Clapp, argued that, "all the niceties of definition are needless if we can say that a physician may in good faith disregard the words of the statute if the health of his patient requires such advice in the same way that he may lawfully perform an abortion—flatly and unconditionally forbidden by statute."[32] Clapp was aware, however, that abortion and birth control might not be interpreted as completely analogous in the strictest legal sense. In the case of abortion, if a woman's life was in danger and she was pregnant, there existed no other option for medical treatment. In the case of birth control, however, Clapp argued that "the condition to be guarded against need not arise if the parties concerned abstain from acting." In contrast to performing an abortion, offering birth control represented a way to "avoid the consequences of an act not yet performed."[33] He warned the League that judges might interpret the laws in a number of different ways depending on the circumstances of each case. Clapp's opinion convinced the League that physicians could not rely on judicial review and, therefore, it began to organize its first campaign for legislative reform.

In November 1929, BCLM secretary Mary East sent a letter to members providing them with the latest news regarding the League's agenda: "The work of the BCLM is processing quietly but steadily. Its chief effort at the present time is to get the medical profession as a whole behind the movement. When the League is strong enough and the demand of physicians general enough the League will go to the legislature to make the law clear and explicit in favor of physicians."[34] Massachusetts doctors did not remain "behind the movement" for long. While both the first BCLM and the FWF addressed their propaganda and educational campaigns to Massachusetts citizens and, in particular, to women who were club members, the new league targeted physicians as the most significant group to recruit to the cause. This orientation would have important consequences for the League throughout the 1930s. Its first priority was to make doctors aware of the ambiguities in the state penal code regarding the prescription of contraceptive materials. Next, it imagined that outraged physicians would lead a charge in the legislature to clarify the laws so that they might practice medicine properly.

Unfortunately, conditions in Massachusetts foisted a legislative campaign on the League before it considered itself ready. Only two months after East had described the BCLM as proceeding quietly and implied that it was not yet strong enough to take on the state legislature, a maverick representative from western Massachusetts introduced a birth control bill in the lower house of the state legislature. East described the situation as an emergency taking place in the form of a legislative battle that "has been thrust upon us."[35] Representative W. Taylor Day of Great Barrington had introduced a bill of his own initiative to encourage the dissemination of birth control information by physicians. East claimed that, as the bill was presently worded, "it may make conditions worse rather than better."[36] Day's actual petition asked that "the Department of Public Health be authorized to register physicians for the purpose of disseminating contraceptive information among married persons," thereby not straying far from the BCLM's stated goals.[37] However, the League considered Day's bill too confrontational, worrying that it would open the floodgates of opposition it sought to quell through its quieter activities. The League wished to avoid any reference to birth control, envisioning a reformed state law that would refer only to physicians' rights to treat their patients without state interference. Ultimately, the BCLM and its physician allies succeeded in persuading Representative Day to withdraw the bill without a hearing. The reformers argued in their annual report that it "seemed wiser to make a fresh start next year than to try to substitute a bill."[38] Thus, by 1930 birth controllers in the state of Massachusetts had yet to make any effort to reform the laws prohibiting the exhibition and dissemination of birth control. Their inactivity throughout the 1920s, however, only served to put them on par with other state leagues, as no state birth control battles were won during this entire decade.

Beginning in 1930, the BCLM made numerous focused efforts to reach out to doctors, offer them support, and recruit them into the League. In her annual report, for example, East wrote that 250 doctors attended a meeting at Ames's home to hear Dr. Robert Dickinson speak on the medical aspects of birth control. At this meeting, "It was voted . . . that a committee of doctors be appointed to find the best procedure under the present law by which contraceptive information could be given for adequate reasons."[39] Thus, the League decided to defer to doctors not only in regard to the best methods of contraception, but also in the arena of politics and strategy. This decision would alter the face of the Massachusetts birth control movement throughout the remainder of the interwar years and beyond.[40]

In 1931 the BCLM and a group of Massachusetts physicians initiated a short-lived and unsuccessful legislative campaign to clarify the exemption of physicians from birth control prohibitions along the lines of the New York state penal code. At the first meeting of the newly established doctors' committee of the BCLM it was decided that physicians would be more comfortable giving contraceptive information to their patients under a modified law, rather than having to rely on favorable judicial interpretation of the existing statutes. The Massachusetts Doctors' Bill of 1931 did not specifically ask that physicians be registered by the Department of Public Health (as Day's bill had done), but petitioned, simply, "to remove the uncertainty in the minds of physicians and their legal advisors as to whether under the existing laws physicians, hospitals, medical schools, etc. are restricted in giving treatment prescriptions and instruction for the protection of health and prevention of disease."[41]

Ames played in integral part in formulating the role the League would play in relation to the Doctor's Bill of 1931. She claimed, first and foremost, that the bill was a doctors' bill and should not be directly associated with the BCLM or the birth control movement at large. She also argued that the bill, as designed by physicians, was a conservative measure attempting merely to clarify the law to avoid the risk of prosecution, rather than creating new legislation. Like East, she advised birth controllers to work quietly in a supportive role to the physicians.

Both East and Ames often used the word "deference" to describe the nature of their relationship to the physicians they had brought into the fray. Ames counseled moderation, imploring birth control reformers to allow doctors to determine publicity, and to avoid religious issues and the criticism of any groups during the duration of the legislative campaign. She argued that birth control propaganda—which she defined as naturally including feminist and economic arguments for the use of contraceptives—should be laid aside for the moment in favor of the more palatable arguments for physicians' legal rights and maternal and infant health.[42]

That Ames believed in a broader reform agenda on a personal level only accentuates the extent to which her alliance with physicians constituted a deliberate political strategy. In a letter whose purpose was to gather support for the state Doctors' Bill, Ames explained the scope and aim of the legislation in this way: "Of all legislation petitioned for in recent years, this is the most vital to women,—not vital in a figurative sense, but vital as a matter of life and death to hundreds of married women yearly in this state. The bill is a conservative measure restricting itself entirely to medical issues. General birth control considerations, the economic, the eugenic, the social betterment lie outside its scope. Its purpose is to prevent physical suffering, disease and death."[43] Ames used seasoned tactics, appealing to people's respect for physicians and their concern for the health of mothers while downplaying the radical associations of the birth control movement. She went on to argue that, "the Doctors' Bill simply makes it possible for married women to get effective contraceptive advice when necessary from physicians, than whom there is no more responsible group."[44] Ames consciously cultivated the appeal of better medicine and better babies in order to make a greater impact than Dennett's concurrent arguments for civil liberties.

Whether or not Ames truly believed in the correctness, compassion, and responsible nature of the medical profession, she held out this ideal to the public in her efforts to fortify and enhance the respectability of the movement. She used the tactic of praising physicians for their heroism and chivalry in their efforts to save and improve women's lives precisely in order to convince them to do so. For example, she wrote that, "There is evidenced in the Doctors' Bill an outstanding act of chivalry that should not go unrecorded. Their petition proves their disinterestedness. They have nothing to gain, on the contrary the preventive measures advocated tend to reduce the number of cases in their care. Thoughtful women all over the State are grateful to them for their unselfish help."[45] The BCLM's acceptance of the chivalry of Massachusetts physicians involved elaborate courting rituals, including traditional "feminine" subservience and deference. An alliance with physicians placed the League in a precarious position whereby gaining the trust and support of doctors meant waiving the "right" to criticize or challenge the noble profession. Ames had to maintain a delicate balance, having at once to court doctors' attention to the issue and then to praise them for their leadership in the struggle. Her plan to exempt physicians from prohibitions regarding birth control required the development of a self-fulfilling prophecy through which Ames projected, provoked, and then graciously accepted physicians' leadership.

In the campaign for the Massachusetts Doctors' Bill, the BCLM eventually questioned once again even the use of the term "birth control" in publicity pamphlets, leaflets, and letters. East wrote to Ames in January 1931 with worries that, if the BCLM used the term "birth control" in a leaflet about the Doctors' Bill, "It will look like one and the same thing and we have taken pains to try to make them look different."[46]

The hearing on the Doctors' Bill (now called Senate Bill No. 43) began at the state house in February 1931. What transpired at the hearings took its supporters by complete surprise. Birth control reformers had falsely begun to believe that, by siding with medicine, science, and public health, they would avoid the turmoil of both religious and political embroilments. This did not turn out to be true. Despite careful strategizing to make the true intent of the Doctor's Bill virtually unrecognizable, the opposition, especially Catholic opposition, recognized the threat and mobilized accordingly.

As Dennett had done on Capitol Hill, Ames placed most, if not all, of the blame for the defeat of the bill on Catholic opposition. In a form letter she wrote immediately after the hearing, Ames's anger and frustration are evident:

> We have all been troubled by the fear that this Catholic threat to our free institutions would materialize if Catholics were given positions of power in our government, but never before in so short a time have events developed in such irrefutable sequence as in this case of opposition to the Doctors' Bill. The opportunity was there to read this bill with understanding of its *medical* nature, but the Roman Church chose to consider it a birth control measure and condemn it on the grounds of degeneracy.[47]

One year before the hearings, Pope Pius XI had codified the Catholic position on birth control in his encyclical "Of Chaste Marriage." In this document, the Pope reinforced prohibitions against infidelity, birth control, divorce, and abortion, thereby disassociating the Roman Catholic church from the liberalizing trends of the Anglican church, the Federal Council of the Churches of Christ in America, and segments of the Jewish community.[48]

In addition to giving the League a glimpse of the strength of Catholic opposition, the defeat of the Massachusetts Doctors' Bill temporarily shook the faith of the BCLM in the power of the medical profession to overcome all obstacles. According to Linda Gordon, the BCLM learned that "no matter how decorous and conservative the League's arguments for birth control, they could not escape redbaiting and other forms of scurrilous attack."[49]

The defeat also uncovered tensions within the organization over its conservative tendencies, for some members now saw this conservatism as an ineffective political strategy. In April 1931, for example, a member resigned from the BCLM over a disagreement about strategy and authority. He had wished to publicize the names of those who signed the petition to pass Senate Bill No. 43, but was rebuffed by the League's board of directors. He responded by criticizing league officers for "always err(ing) on the side of squeamishness."[50] Ames responded to this resignation with a defense of the decision makers in the BCLM, based on the difficulty of their position. After all, she argued, "Senate bill number 43 was in fact a doctors' bill and not a general birth control measure and their wishes had to be considered in every move we made if we were to be of real help to them and to maintain their confidence in us."[51] If there was squeamishness in the League's position, Ames claimed that it could be explained as a "squeamish regard for the point of view of the physicians."[52] Ames's answer to the disgruntled member revealed her recognition of the tendencies he complained about, but an unwillingness to break free from the League's obligations. These tensions continued to plague the League throughout the 1930s, making it less capable of handling an increasingly bleak political situation.

Ultimately, the BCLM's affiliation with physicians continued in spite of the defeat of Senate Bill No. 43. Ames counted herself among the conservatives who endorsed this policy. In 1931, she wrote to the supporters of the bill to assure them that her organization "stands ready to carry on and cooperate with the doctors in every legal effort to bring help to sick women who may be victims of death and disease if deprived of medical aid."[53] Thus, Ames continued to make her organization available to

Massachusetts's doctors. She also continued to remind physicians that there existed no restriction against giving oral information about birth control in the hope that, while the laws were in the process of changing, women in Massachusetts could obtain the information and contraception they needed from their doctors. Thus, Ames found herself navigating her organization through treacherous waters as she had done in the immediate postwar years, again counseling pragmatism over boldness. However, new legal and economic considerations would soon embolden Ames, offering her an opportunity to bring her political agenda closer to her personal beliefs.

RELYING ON JUDGES/DEFYING SANGER

When the League obtained a new legal opinion that interpreted the state penal code in a very favorable way, it changed courses once again. In 1932, legal counselor Murray F. Hall argued that it followed logically from decided cases that, "A physician is justified in giving contraceptive advice for the purpose of saving life, safeguarding health or preventing disease." He went on to claim that a physician "may give such advice whenever the condition of the patient would warrant the performance of a therapeutic abortion if she were pregnant or would justify sterilization."[54] Hall's opinion convinced Ames and the executive board that the BCLM could rely on favorable interpretations of existing state laws rather than trying to engage in a difficult legislative battle. After the disappointing experience in the state house only one year earlier, Ames was relieved that the League would not be forced to go head-to-head with conservative legislators and Catholic activists.

Hall's opinion was quite encouraging in that it offered the most favorable interpretation of the state penal code that the BCLM could have hoped for. He went so far as to assert that state statutes, "do not purport to regulate in any way the practice of physicians and should not be held to apply to physicians who are in the *bona fide* practice of their professions."[55] The BCLM took heart and decided to give up its legislative efforts, instead working to promote the novel (and as yet untested) idea that physicians could legally prescribe contraceptives to their married patients for health reasons in the state of Massachusetts. In a letter to league members, Ames described this new work as simply giving Massachusetts physicians "further confidence."[56] This work was not so simple, however, and doctors turned out to be a harder sell than the BCLM anticipated. Only one year before, the BCLM had convinced physicians that they needed clarification of state laws to practice medicine without fear of prosecution. Now the League reversed its position and tried to convince these same physicians that the present laws presented no danger to them.

One of the ways the BCLM attempted to give physicians more confidence to prescribe birth control was by downplaying the legal prohibitions against this practice in its propaganda. Ames expressed concern that physicians were not aware of their rights and were being bullied into silence by the specter of the federal Comstock Laws. This worry represented a complete reversal for Ames, as her earlier public relations strategy had emphasized the peculiar disadvantage under which Massachusetts physicians worked. For example, in a letter from the fall of 1931, Ames had asserted, "Massachusetts mothers lack the medical protection which is available in over forty other states. Massachusetts physicians are handicapped in giving aid which would preserve the health and often save the lives of their patients."[57] By 1932 Ames changed her tune and argued that "physicians throughout the nation have been led to believe erroneously that contraceptive aid to their patients is illegal under state statutes and court decisions."[58] Ames now asserted that doctors' fear of prescribing birth control was based on a misinterpretation of the law. She claimed that, "if physicians can be made to realize that the giving of such aid in the bona fide practice of their profession is definitely *not* illegal, the greatest obstacle confronting us will be removed," thereby dismissing Comstock and state statutes as obstacles.[59]

In complete contrast to both Sanger and Dennett (and her own earlier convictions), Ames came to argue that neither federal nor state laws constituted a real threat to Massachusetts physicians. This position was to become a point of contention between Ames and Sanger throughout the 1930s. Specifically, Ames criticized Sanger for overestimating the power of the Comstock Law to control physicians, overgeneralizing from the national case and thereby discouraging doctors in her own state from prescribing birth control. In a letter to Sanger, Ames argued, "It is not a correct conception of reality under the present circumstances to ignore all the Federal Court decisions and the Postal Rulings . . . and put in print that there are no exceptions under Sections 211, 245, 311, 312, of the U.S. Penal Code."[60] In a speech before the Chicago Woman's City Club, Ames made a similar argument: "The legal situation in Massachusetts has been generally misunderstood. The statutes are not clear in wording. They have been misinterpreted, and false statements of their meaning have been printed in important works on birth control with many harmful results."[61] The critical reference to important printed works on birth control can only have meant Dennett's *Birth Control Laws* (published in 1926), which certainly painted the Massachusetts picture as bleak. Thus, Ames's decision in 1932 to rely on judicial review alienated her from Dennett as well as Sanger.

Because of Ames's resentment of Sanger's overzealous and supposedly misdirected propaganda campaign, she refused to cooperate with her campaign to reform federal legislation. In a 1934 letter to Sanger, Ames argued that recent letters between the BCLM and postal authorities "confirm our belief that the federal statutes hold only within their scope prohibitions of unworthy actions based on unworthy motives."[62] She claimed that Sanger interpreted the federal law in the strictest manner and that judicial interpretations were likely to be more liberal and take intent into consideration. Despite what historians have portrayed as Sanger's almost mystical authority over birth control reformers in the interwar years, Ames and her league directly challenged Sanger's justification for tackling federal legislative reform.

> As I interpret these rulings . . . they show that those are mistaken who maintain that no exemptions exist under the present wording of the Federal Statutes. . . . Court decisions, plus medical practice, plus popular education, have created rights and privileges under the law which could easily be lost through legislative tinkering with the Federal Statues and might make it necessary to undertake legislative changes in the state laws. For Massachusetts that is an impossible task.[63]

Thus, Ames no longer viewed Sanger's federal efforts as compatible with her own, but, rather, as a direct, if unwitting, threat. The BCLM now disassociated itself not only from Sanger's federal campaign, but from legislative reform at the state level as well.

Hall's opinion had convinced Ames that women in Massachusetts as well as women throughout the nation could place their health and their families in the hands of sympathetic doctors and judges. This opinion gave the League the strength to stand up to Sanger and even question her judgment. In this same letter dated May 1934, the author (probably East) asked, "Doesn't some way open by which you can get out of this Federal legislation jam? Is there anything we can do to help? Mrs. Ames and I would like to be with you one hundred percent but if you feel you have to keep pegging away at the federal legislation in its present form, how could we be so?"[64]

Sanger reacted furiously to Ames's and East's challenge to her authority. She mocked their optimism and naïveté and charged them with expecting her to "lay down arms and be satisfied with a flimsy ruling based on the case of a venereal man and a tubercular woman."[65] The

Massachusetts women countered that their criticism was "not against changing the Federal Statutes wisely, but is directed against the form and content of your amendment on the grounds that it is restrictive of our existing liberties and could be a source of oppression in the future."[66] Ames was convinced that interpretations of existing state laws would prove more permissive than Sanger's proposed federal legislation. Ames's two points of contention with Sanger were, first, Sanger's use of what Ames deemed "scare tactics" to make physicians unduly anxious about prescribing birth control, and, second, Sanger's assumption that her reform strategy would work for everyone. Ames objected to the federal bill Sanger supported because it limited the receipt and distribution of contraceptive materials to physicians and licensed clinics. According to Ames, "Licenses are issued by the states and it is highly improbable that we could secure a license for such a clinic in this state."[67] Thus, Sanger's focus on federal matters was read as insensitivity to the situation in the state of Massachusetts. In addition, Ames claimed that Sanger advanced conflicting arguments. As Ames saw it, on the one hand, Sanger argued that clinics were illegal under present laws; on the other, she actively solicited funds for the opening of clinics. Ames even implied that she was less than confident of Sanger's integrity when she pointed out that Sanger never accounted for funds she received. Therefore, the BCLM would offer no further money to her organization.

Ames's growing rift with Sanger developed out of a new confidence bolstered by legal opinions and court decisions that provided evidence that Comstock was surmountable.

> The rulings I obtained were necessary for us to prove to our physicians and advisors that these statutes and others you have sent out are not in conformity with the law nor the customary practice of Postal Authorities, and that neither the physicians nor their hospitals and clinics need fear Federal interference. I maintain that misinformation about the law, rousing false fear among the medical fraternity is detrimental to the work of birth control and of vital danger.[68]

Ames's criticism of Sanger echoed the earlier words of Mary Dennett. Dennett had also rejected Sanger's early rhetoric as alienating and antagonistic to politicians. Moreover, Dennett decried Sanger's tendency toward the dramatic, arguing that Sanger's desire for personal aggrandizement meant that she characterized every situation as grave and every scuffle as a great battle. Years later, Ames found fault with Sanger's "rousing false fears" among the physicians whose confidence she sought to bolster.

Both women charged Sanger with making a political situation worse through her confrontational style.

Continuing its policy since its first incarnation in 1916 of following the path of least resistance and avoiding controversy, the BCLM now had at its disposal a legal opinion to reinforce its trepidation regarding legislative reform. But by the mid-thirties the BCLM had worked itself into a problematic situation. Dominated by conservative members who wanted the League to maintain its association with physicians and avoid legislative activity, it still faced the reticence of Massachusetts doctors to make this cause their own. Understandably, many physicians were likely suspicious of the assurances offered by the League, as they reflected such a marked contrast from its earlier propaganda. Trouble with physicians and with Sanger forced the League to reformulate its agenda once again by the mid-thirties. With the depression raging and the very survival of women and children at stake, Ames fashioned a new agenda designed to get birth control information and materials into the hands of the women in her state.

THE DEPRESSION: CLINICS, COURTS, AND THE RESIGNATION OF AMES

Instead of undertaking political reform and grappling proactively with reticence among Massachusetts physicians to carry out research or a legislative campaign, the BCLM embarked on new strategies in the 1930s. Relying on Hall's opinion that assumed the legality of physician-supervised birth control dissemination, and responding to the great misery produced by the economic depression, Ames convinced the League to open up birth control clinics in Massachusetts. These "Mothers' Health Offices" (MHOs) would be places where married women could receive contraceptive advice and materials for medical reasons under the supervision of licensed physicians.[69] The new commitment to clinics was ripe with ironies and unintended consequences. Initiated by a conservative state league in the face of inauspicious political circumstances, the clinics would ultimately radicalize and derail the movement in Massachusetts: they would encourage reformers to push for a broader set of indications for legitimate use of birth control in the face of women's real needs as clinic patients, and they would provoke judicial test cases that placed the state of Massachusetts in the unenviable position of being the sole state that prohibited physicians from prescribing birth control to their patients.

Ames was moved by the depression to abandon her long-standing commitment to conservatism and marketing birth control solely as a medical issue. Like many birth control reformers in the 1930s, she began to use economic arguments to promote her cause. However, important distinctions existed between those who promoted birth control as a measure of fiscal conservatism and those who promoted it as a way to mitigate human suffering. Ames was aligned with the latter group, while many other powerful members of the BCLM and the ABCL were aligned with the former.[70]

In the early 1930s Ames, for the first time, acknowledged publicly the economic advantages of birth control. Rather than promoting birth control as a panacea that would make social welfare expenditures unnecessary, Ames sought cooperation with New Deal agencies. In 1934, for example, Ames sent three hundred letters to directors of various welfare committees offering them the names of doctors who would provide contraceptives "for medical reasons and . . . for economic reasons because of the existing emergency."[71] Ames wanted birth control to become a part of the nation's relief and welfare efforts and complained when the League was not allowed to participate in the Emergency Relief Drive because officials "felt that our organization is 'of a somewhat different character.'"[72] This response, although typical, was particularly frustrating to Ames who, since 1916, had taken great pains to promote birth control as a mainstream and respectable social welfare cause.

Harkening back to the rhetoric of the immediate postwar period, Ames began to call attention to the obvious links between fertility control and maternal and infant health. However, in this period, state-sponsored social welfare programs were growing rather than shrinking; Ames's more confident tone reflects this context. In a letter asking for contributions for the League's MHOs, Ames capitalized on concerns about high maternal mortality rates: "The Birth Control League is the only organization which seeks to lessen Massachusetts' share of these appalling losses by control of the original cause, that is, through the postponement of pregnancy until the mother's health is adequate for the task of pregnancy and labor."[73] Ames tried to encourage the public to view birth control as a part of a larger relief effort. In the face of rejection by federal relief agencies, Ames argued that birth control "gets at the root of many of the evils that you are helping to combat at much greater expense through the charitable agencies."[74] Thus, she linked past and present concerns and rhetoric—promoting birth control as a maternalist cause and touting its economic benefits.

Part of the problem the BCLM faced in seeking inclusion in national welfare programs was strong opposition by Katharine Lenroot, the chief of the CB. After the passage of the Social Security Act in 1935, the

Bureau regained some of the authority and power it had lost in the late 1920s when Sheppard-Towner was deprived of its appropriations. Now the Bureau would be responsible for administering Title Five of the Social Security Act. Based to a large degree on Sheppard-Towner, Title Five provided federal funds for maternal and child health services. Although the Bureau had itself conducted innovative studies that proved the direct association between infant mortality and number of children, space between children, and family income, it had remained—mostly for political reasons—opposed to birth control. According to one of her employees in the Bureau, Lenroot objected to the Bureau's taking on the "extra hazards involved in the acceptance of its programs by administratively assuming responsibility for an activity which is . . . controversial. . . ."[75] Thus, the birth controllers found themselves unable to rely on the most powerful, female-run federal bureau to initiate a program that promised to substantially lower maternal and infant mortality. Ironically, this decision on the part of the Bureau was based on the same kind of political pragmatism and timidity that had shaped the policies of the BCLM since its creation in 1916.

Ames clearly saw birth control as a way to improve the circumstances of people's lives, rather than merely a way to save money. In contrast to some in her cohort Ames's compassion for poor women was never overshadowed by her fear of the growth of the "dependent classes." In a letter to women welfare directors she wrote, "These times must make you realize only too clearly the tragedy that the conception of another child would bring to the unemployed mother upon whose shoulders falls the support of the family. *These women, haunted by the fear of another pregnancy, are entitled to instruction in the control of contraception. They have a right to it.*"[76] Far from leading her to condemn the irresponsible spike in the number of welfare babies, the depression encouraged Ames to define birth control as a right of women. This shift in perspective moved her further away from the conservative posture she had struck for many years as president of the League.

Both Ames and Dennett became more "rights-oriented" as the mainstream movement began to embrace eugenics, fiscal conservatism, and population control in the 1930s and 1940s. Ames's commitment to the right of all classes of married women to obtain birth control led to a major conflict with her colleagues in the larger movement and in her own league. As with Dennett, her emerging "rights orientation" underscored violations of individual rights so characteristic of the movement in the 1930s.

On January 5, 1935, the *Boston Transcript* ran an advertisement for the BCLM that read:

TAXPAYERS! Nearly a quarter of a million children were born last year to families entirely supported by you through public relief. Our organization exists to help those parents have only those many children as they can support. Will You Help Us Do This Preventive Work? Contributions may be sent to our office. . . .[77]

Ames was so disturbed by the implications of such publicity that she resigned as president of the League later that year. Writing to the executive committee of the BCLM, she launched a serious critique of the advertisement:

The advertisement in the hands of . . . any opponent of birth control is a weapon with which we can be attacked again and again. In it, our appeal for support is not based on broad humanitarian motives, but is based on the motive of saving money alone. . . . it implies coercion: it may be interpreted to mean restriction of birth by abortion, or sterilization. Voluntary regulation of conception is our idea, isn't it?[78]

Cornelia James Cannon, the League's vice president, mounted a strong defense of the advertisement in which she ignored Ames's important distinction between a coercive and a voluntary program. In the face of this, Ames clarified her objections to the advertisement. Her objections fell into two categories: first, the advertisement misstated economic facts, and, second, it distorted the true aims of the League. Claiming that nearly one-quarter of a million children were being entirely supported by Massachusetts taxpayers was a gross oversimplification and overgeneralization. Ames argued that depression records were so at variance as to make reliable statistics impossible to find. In addition, she objected that their organization existed to help parents have only as many children as they *want*, or want to support, rather than "as many as they can support," as the advertisement read. Ames stated her position more fully to Cannon when she wrote, "The object we seek goes through the medical, beyond the economic aspects even, and **strives to protect the personal freedom of the individual** to get adequate contraceptive aid, and to leave her free from control by self-appointed judges who seek to determine for her what are proper motives."[79] Ames's disavowal of the "self-appointed judges" of women could have had various referents: federal and state judges, Roman Catholics, physicians, welfare workers, or even middle-class and elite birth control reformers who sought control over the reproductive choices of poor women. This letter marked the first time Ames officially stated—even within her own organization—that she advocated contraceptive use for purely personal reasons. Within four years, she had made a huge leap from advocating a purely medical agenda to one that encompassed economic and individual indicators for family planning. While throughout the teens and twenties her nascent boldness could be surmised in her writings and the observations of others, the economic crisis and the League's response to it had made it manifest. She had moved from consciously limiting the parameters of the movement for pragmatic reasons to allowing her ethical commitments to guide her positions outside the mainstream.

Like Dennett, Ames objected to being associated with racist eugenists who sought to sterilize the "unfit" and encourage the birth rate among the "correct" classes of people. She had witnessed the national movement deteriorate into "a conservative program of social control," through which the middle classes could be spared the expense and discomfort of living among undesirables by limiting their fertility.[80] Linda Gordon has argued that the 1920s and 1930s witnessed "birth controllers' conversion to eugenics and their desertion of feminism."[81] Most historians agree that this tendency was clearly evident in the ABCL and among state leagues as well. For example, the Pennsylvania Birth Control Federation printed an even more straightforward advertisement in the mid-1930s that actually calculated the state's cost of keeping alive an unwanted child for three weeks. The headline read, "Nobody Wanted Jimmy . . . But He Was Born Anyhow . . . And Died Three Weeks Later." It went on to say that neither Jimmy's parents nor his community wanted him but that, after adding the cost of prenatal care, hospital costs, and burial costs, the dead infant cost the taxpayers of Pennsylvania over $300.[82] Ames's reaction to the advertising campaign in 1935 must be seen in the context of this national trend. Always conscious of the connections between maternal and infant welfare and birth control, Ames remained dedicated to a movement that championed reproductive reform rather than fiscal conservativism.

In a letter to members of the BCLM written three weeks after the publicity controversy, Ames would not let the incident rest:

> That advertisement was open to fair criticism on several grounds. In the first place it did not do justice to the true motives of the League, because it was an appeal to Taxpayers as a class on the basis of protecting their pocketbooks, rather than an appeal to all citizens on the basis of rendering genuine service to all our people, rich and poor, taxpayers and non-taxpayers.[83]

Ames also objected to the "harsh and inhumane" emphasis of the piece. She feared that the public might get the impression that the League "aimed at denying parents the joys and compensations of parenthood merely because they are poor."[84]

Ames's decision to distance herself from the right wing of the birth control or eugenics movement by emphasizing voluntary family limitation did not represent a full turning away from her commitment to practical politics. The publicity controversy of 1935 also brought to the surface some tensions in the BCLM regarding the constitution of the League as it related to authority and decision making. A combination of these two issues led Ames to resign as the League's president in 1935.

In contrast to the position she took regarding the controversial advertisement, when it came to the working of the League Ames found herself pitted against a group whom she perceived as being "full of revolutionary ideas."[85] Angered that the ad was published without her knowledge or approval, Ames worried about a lack of structure in the League and came down squarely on the side of law and order. She wrote,

> I understand the restlessness of an ardent spirit curbed by old rules and old promises or contracts. But these contracts are actualities. Our agreements with doctors, the Mothers Health Office, and our League Members are binding on us. . . . Now if certain members of the Executive Committee or members of the League don't feel that they can subscribe to the Constitution and the contracts existing between the League and its Advisory Board, its doctor members and League members, then those members should withdraw and form the kind of new organization that does suit them . . . in which they can do just as they please.[86]

Ames reminded League members that they were "tied hand and foot by binding agreements with other groups—ministers, doctors, professors, Advisory Council, etc" and that these groups needed to be consulted before the BCLM moved in new and potentially damaging directions.

As Ames was beginning to broaden her own view of legitimate indications for the use of birth control, her relations with Sanger and her own league became strained. On the one hand, she continued to fight vigorously in her own state against dramatic propaganda that would dissuade physicians from cooperating with the League. On the other hand, she complained to Sanger that her federal bill would amount to a medical monopoly over birth control information and that it left out economic or social reasons for family limitation. In a letter to Sanger in June 1934, Ames made clear her personal trepidation regarding reliance on the medical community, a dependency that she took pains to cover up among Massachusetts birth control reformers:

Under your proposed amendment we would be as much at the caprice of the doctors and their medical associates as we have been in the past. *We still would be apologizing supplicants on the medical doorstep.* . . . An organized campaign by the doctors and one determining vote at their annual meeting could put out of the reach of women all contraceptive aid in that community. Men and women would be deprived by Federal amendment of receiving by mail . . . any knowledge or materials on contraception from any source other than doctors. Freedom of access to scientific discoveries should not be made by statute the property of the medical profession alone. Such an arrangement smacks of the privileges accorded to the 'medicine man' of old.[87]

Indeed, as this letter illustrates, by the mid-1930s Ames's position regarding federal legislation was closer to Dennett's than to Sanger's. As the previous chapter has shown, this shift of opinion was shared by others in the movement who were increasingly attracted to Dennett's formulation of the issue rather than Sanger's. Ames's evolving position grew out of her increasing concern for women's health during the crisis of the Great Depression as well as optimism engendered by that same crisis. Ames's optimism regarding the eventual acceptance of birth control, however, did not extend to Dennett's faith that relief would come through the legislative process.

In 1935, just as Ames began to waffle in her position regarding the power of the medical profession, economic and personal indicators for birth control use, and the distinction between state and federal strategies, she resigned as president of the BCLM. A major reason for her resignation was the publicity controversy that pitted her authority against other members of the executive board. She had been the leader of the birth control movement in Massachusetts since its inception in 1916. Problems like the one engendered by the advertisement in the *Transcript* called into question her ability to lead the movement. In addition, Ames's disagreements with Sanger continued, as did her discomfort with the increasing influence of eugenic, population control, and anti–New Deal sentiment in the birth control movement. She was unable to face the conundrum she herself had created, that is, how to mesh her political decision to promote birth control on the coattails of the powerful medical profession with her own strong belief in the broader implications of the movement. Indeed, the struggle to find a solution to this particular puzzle would continue to plague the BCLM throughout the 1930s.

Abandoning the frustrating and complex arena of legislation, the League began the work of establishing clinics.[88] Ames saw this effort as a

way to work with and under the direction of physicians while also expanding the number of married women who would be eligible to receive birth
control information. She explained this strategy in a letter to a fellow
member. "Four years ago," she wrote, "the doctors tried to introduce an
amendment to these sections of the law which would make clear the right
of physicians to advise. Like most attempts to change such section of law
by legislative action, it failed. It was then decided to open a MHO, where
advice would be given under this more liberal interpretation of the law."[89]
Ames went on to say that, to date, Sanger's clinics and the BCLM's own
MHOs still demanded medical indications to disseminate birth control.
Ames committed herself to changing this policy to include economic indications, arguing that, "As yet poverty is not accepted as a medical indication
at our Health Offices. The entire Board thinks it should be and every effort
is being made to bring our doctors and lawyers to this point of view."[90]

     This development in the BCLM mirrored the ABCL during the same
period, as both organizations turned toward creating clinics as a less controversial and more effective strategy than attempting legislative reform.[91]
Inspired by the economic suffering brought on by the depression, birth
controllers exhibited a renewed interest in practical action and provision-
ary strategies. The move to establish clinics also reflected a growing recognition that legislative reform was not only time-consuming, but hadn't
yielded any positive results in approximately twenty years. Thus, both
political and economic circumstances shaped new tactics. Massachusetts
reformers, like their national counterparts, sought the path of least resistance to get birth control materials into the hands of American women.

     By 1936 the BCLM had clinics in Brookline (1932), Springfield
(1934), Worcester (1935), and Salem (1936). By the end of the next year,
three more opened in Boston's South End, New Bedford, and Fitchburg.
These achievements came in the wake of the *U.S. v. One Package* decision
in 1936, and the endorsement of birth control by the AMA in 1937. In
U.S. v. One Package, Judge Hand of the U.S. Circuit Court of Appeals sustained the ruling of the District Court that birth control literature and
devices imported for use by physicians were not restricted by federal
obscenity statutes. Hand ruled that it was not the purpose of federal
statutes to interfere with conscientious medical practices. When the U.S.
Attorney General announced that the government would rest its case, the
decision became, in effect, the law. After the *One Package* decision, the
U.S. Treasury Department issued instructions to customs authorities to
admit birth control supplies addressed to physicians.

     In 1937 the AMA finally recognized birth control as a legitimate part
of medical practice. This admission manifested itself in the coordination

of the ABCL and Sanger's Clinical Research Bureau into a united Birth
Control Federation of America. According to one historian, the AMA
had little choice by the end of the 1930s but to accept birth control so that
it could control its dissemination. "Demand for contraceptives out-
stripped the supply of medical knowledge and gave rise to a huge birth
control industry riddled with quackery and dishonesty," and, therefore,
doctors found it necessary to proceed with research and dissemination.[92]
By the end of the 1930s, with federal court cases decided in their favor and
the acceptance of birth control by the AMA, birth control reformers felt
confident that their worries could be put to rest. Indeed, it seemed that
birth control was finally becoming an acceptable and accepted practice, at
least among married couples. While most birth controllers were satisfied
with these victories, Dennett and Ames remained critical of the restrictions
that American women seeking to control their fertility still encountered.
Incidents in Massachusetts in the late 1930s would make clear the extent
of the limitations placed on the dissemination and use of birth control.

POST-AMES'S PRESIDENCY, POST—*ONE PACKAGE* EVENTS IN MASSACHUSETTS

By 1937, armed with new confidence, members of the BCLM were prepared "to make every effort to broaden the classification of women who
may be accepted in Health Offices."[93] With the AMA and the federal
government on its side, and with no end in sight to the economic depression, the BCLM began to believe that it could stretch the law in order to
accommodate economic reasons for family limitation. Although the
League's lawyer did not believe that birth control reformers could rely on
favorable interpretation of statutes in the case of dissemination based on
economic factors, one member wrote, "It is difficult for me to believe that
we would not get a favorable decision for a case of this sort."[94] No one in
the BCLM could have anticipated the setbacks that visited the movement
in Massachusetts in the summer of 1937.

In June 1937, police raided the BCLM's North Shore MHO. They
confiscated all records and charged Dr. Lucile Lord Heinstein, a nurse, and
two social workers with exhibiting, advertising, and selling birth control. In
July all four were indicted in the District Court of Salem, where Judge
Sears ruled that it was indeed illegal for physicians to provide birth control
information to ill, married women. The case was appealed to the Superior
Court of Essex County in the fall of 1937. The BCLM believed that the
Superior Court would "not sustain a ruling which does not recognize that

the Massachusetts law aims at indecency and is not intended to interfere with a medical practice approved by the AMA."[95] By October, however, Superior Court Judge Wilford Gray upheld the earlier conviction and found all four MHO workers guilty of selling and giving away articles for contraception. In its press release, the BCLM tried to sound optimistic. It argued that Judge Gray was sympathetic to the defendants and therefore released them and imposed a minimum fine of $100 apiece. The League felt confident that the next step, appealing the case before the Supreme Court of Massachusetts, would bring successful results. Judge Gray had implied that he did not wish to take the authority and responsibility for interpreting the statutes in question in a new way, for this duty was more properly in the purview of the Supreme Court or the legislature.[96] Before the case came to the Supreme Court in 1938, two other MHOs were raided in Brookline and the South End.

When the appeal to the Superior Court failed to bring positive results, the BCLM attempted to re-engage the activism of doctors around the issue of their professional rights and privileges. It sent a letter to members of the Massachusetts Medical Society in October 1937 informing them of "a grave situation" that had arisen in Massachusetts. They were told that physicians' rights had been violated, "First, in the seizure and holding of confidential medical records by the police; second by police interference with the right of physicians to practice medicine in accordance with accepted methods."[97] The BCLM urged physicians to endorse an enclosed statement of protest in the hope that, as in the case of New York in 1929, concerted protest by physicians would be "of great value in establishing the fact that contraception was a part of sound medical practice rather than an indecency."[98]

The situation in Massachusetts did arouse the interest and concern of physicians at large. When the MHO workers were first found guilty in July, an editorial appeared in the *New England Journal of Medicine*. This editorial argued that the prohibitions in Massachusetts were no more drastic than the federal Comstock Laws, which the U.S. Circuit Court of Appeals had already interpreted as exempting doctors in the *One Package* decision one year earlier. Therefore, there should be no question that physicians were not lawbreakers when they administered or offered contraceptive materials to save lives or to promote the health of their patients. The editorial went on to argue that the AMA "has expressed itself only in regard to relation of physician and patient," and that its approval of contraception should not "be construed as favoring the use of such measures for the solution of social problems."[99] The author then praised the BCLM in particular for advocating these conservative goals and methods. He claimed that, because birth control reformers in Massachusetts "have apparently respected this limitation to medical indications, . . . they are entitled to the sympathy and support of the medical profession in their present legal difficulties."[100] Thus, Ames's steadfast counsel to the League to uphold its commitments to physicians and defer to their judgment seemed to have paid off. In its time of crisis, the BCLM could rely on the medical profession for support.

The clinic raids and indictments seemed to catalyze not only support but also opposition to birth control in Massachusetts. In October, for instance, Leslie Hawkridge and Caroline Davis of the BCLM were found guilty by the Municipal Court of Boston for distributing written information as to where contraceptive information might be obtained. Ironically, as the rest of the nation began to trust that the movement had passed through its most trying stages, reformers in Massachusetts were just beginning to face the consequences of a conservative political climate and their miscalculations in political strategy. The BCLM found itself at the mercy of what seemed to be the only courts in the country that were willing to prosecute physicians for disseminating birth control for health reasons.

In May 1938, Judge C. J. Rugg of the Massachusetts Supreme Court also found the defendants at the North Shore MHO guilty. His opinion, in *Commonwealth v. Gardner*, illustrates the problem with relying on favorable judicial interpretation rather than legislative reform. The Supreme Court of Massachusetts ruled that the "sale of contraceptives to married women, even on prescription of a physician and for the preservation of life and health according to sound and generally accepted medical practice, is a violation of G.L. (Terr. Ed.) c. 272, and 21."[101] The defendants claimed that they were acting on their attorneys' advice that the statute in question did not apply to articles intended for the use of contraception "upon prescription by a duly qualified physician when necessary for the preservation of life or health according to sound and generally accepted medical practice."[102] Rugg countered that the terms of the statutes in question were "plain, unequivocal and peremptory." He went on to add, "They contain no exceptions. They are sweeping, absolute, and devoid of ambiguity. They are directed with undeviating explicitness against the prevention of conception by any of the means specified. It would be difficult to select appropriate legislative words to express the thought with greater emphasis."[103] Rugg argued that, if the legislature had so wished, it could have easily expressed its intention to provide exemptions or exceptions to the law, as it did in the state of New York, where "physicians are permitted by statute to prescribe contraceptives under limited and defined circumstances."[104] Unlike the case in New York, Rugg argued that there was no evidence to indicate that the Massachusetts legislature had intended to exempt physicians from its prohibitions regarding birth control and it was the duty of the judicial branch to uphold the intention of lawmakers. Rugg went so far as to claim that, "We think such an exception cannot be read into our statute by judicial interpretation. Our statute must be interpreted and enforced as enacted. . . . The relief here urged must be sought from the law-making department and not from the judicial department of government."[105] With this last sentence, Rugg undermined what had been the BCLM's political strategy for almost two decades. He told reformers that the relief they sought would have to come from the legislature, not the courts.

The *Gardner* decision took the BCLM by surprise. It had relied on the exemption of physicians from birth control prohibitions, as had reformers nationally and in other states. All across the country, birth control reformers had discontinued their activities after *U.S. v. One Package,* confident that old laws would now be interpreted in new ways to accommodate modern sensibilities and economic realities. Only in Massachusetts did the strategy seem to be backfiring. In a press release immediately following Justice Rugg's ruling, the League stated,

> The adverse decision of the Massachusetts Supreme Court in the Birth Control case will come as a shock to hundreds of citizens interested in human welfare and public health. The court was given the opportunity to free physicians from doubt as to whether a law clearly aimed at obscenity and immorality should prevent them from legitimate use of a branch of medicine approved by the highest medical authorities. . . . Contraception in the hands of the medical profession is accepted by laws in most civilized countries of the world except those under dictatorship. . . . Only in Massachusetts have the rights of physicians been attacked, and in failing to except the practice of medicine from indecency laws the Supreme Court has lost a chance to bring Massachusetts abreast of a more Enlightened world.[106]

The press release continued by emphasizing the important role that family limitation could play in relieving the suffering of ill health and poverty. It ended on a dramatic note by underscoring the isolation of Massachusetts: "This decision will confirm the general opinion that we, here, are living in the dark ages."[107]

In response to Judge Rugg's decision, the BCLM organized a conference to discuss the possibility of an appeal to the U.S. Supreme Court. The conference participants included the highest officers and the lawyers of the BCLM, along with Sanger and the attorney for the ABCL. The

conference report announced a unanimous vote to appeal to the U.S.
Supreme Court. The attorneys advised reformers that the case could get
to the Supreme Court "on the grounds that in forbidding physicians to
give contraceptives to sick women our statute violates the Fourteenth
Amendment of the Federal Constitution, which read that no state shall
'deprive any person of life, liberty, or property without due process of
law.'"[108] It was also determined that an amicus curiae brief would be filed
on behalf of physicians "to argue solely against the infringement of the
right of physicians which Justice Rugg's decision permits."[109]

In October 1938, the U.S. Supreme Court dismissed the appeal in the
Massachusetts birth control case on the grounds that it failed to raise a
substantial federal question. The BCLM now found itself in a formidable
predicament. A memorandum in November summed its difficult situation as follows:

> As a result of the raids on the League's MHOs in 1937, and the subsequent
> refusal of the U.S. Supreme Court . . . to consider the constitutionality of
> the Massachusetts statute, all clinics are closed and all doctors are "legally"
> prohibited from giving mothers contraceptive materials. The general con-
> sensus seems to show first, that there is little hope of having the law re-
> interpreted . . . ; second, there is little chance of getting the legislature itself
> to amend the law because it is so predominantly Catholic; and third, pub-
> lic opinion is not thoroughly aroused to permit much hope . . . to getting
> the law amended by having the issue placed on the ballot.[110]

Thus, at every turn the BCLM encountered daunting obstacles. The
League was running out of options and pessimism hung over the future of
the movement in Massachusetts. One league officer recommended the initiation of an intensive education campaign directed toward the general public and the organization of doctors and laypeople in an effort to amend the
present laws. Recommended procedures included the initiation of new
court cases, a media campaign that would include newspapers, magazines,
radio, speeches, meetings, films, and dramatized skits to educate the public,
and, finally, a Citizens' Committee for Birth Control made up of outstanding members of the community. While court cases were still considered an
option, this memo also recommended that a petition be initiated in 1940 in
support of the right to vote on whether to amend the present law. In order
to accomplish this end, the Citizens Committee would have to get at least
25,000 signatures on a petition to put pressure on representatives.

At the Eighteenth Annual Meeting of the ABCL in January 1939,
Mrs. Caroline Davis of the BCLM stated that "this Commonwealth

holds the unenviable position of being the only one of the forty-eight states in which an old indecency statute has been interpreted as forbidding physicians to avail themselves of an accepted medical procedure."[111] Birth controllers were not the only group concerned about the unenviable position of the Commonwealth. In January 1939, the *New England Journal of Medicine* again ran an editorial that commented on the sorry state of affairs in Massachusetts. The author claimed that Massachusetts was the only state that interfered with medical advice and practice. He argued that, "These rulings affect not alone marital happiness, the health of women and the well-being of children, but even more fundamentally, they strike at the right of the individual physician to use his knowledge for the benefit of his patients."[112]

By March 1939, the BCLM announced a new outlook and yet another "rebirth" of the League. Just as, twenty years earlier, it sent notice to its members of its decision to become the Family Welfare Foundation, it now claimed once again that, "We have outgrown our old work."[113] The League simultaneously evoked a feeling of optimism about future endeavors and pointed to the futility of its old agenda in the face of state laws and judicial decisions that have "turned back the clock of preventive medicine by fifty years."[114] The League was once again attempting to rally public opinion by broadening the scope of its agenda. It would do so by focusing on the public health benefits of contraception, or "By making apparent the lack of medical contraception in an otherwise well-rounded health program, we will bring home to the citizens of Massachusetts the fact that only in this state are mothers denied this vital aid in planning for tomorrow's children."[115] One month after the declaration of its rebirth, the BCLM announced its new name, "The Massachusetts Mothers' Health Council." This new organization planned to "educate our fellow citizens to see that a sound public health program must begin at the beginning—with the birth of healthy children to well mothers."[116] Since World War I, then, the birth control campaign in Massachusetts had come full circle.

Its new public health agenda brought certain advantages. Worries about the spread of venereal disease and the public acceptance of condoms ultimately came together to work on behalf of the beleaguered Massachusetts birth control movement. In 1940, the BCLM and the married women of Massachusetts received long-awaited relief in the form of the decision of the state supreme court in *Commonwealth v. Corbett*. With Justice Rugg no longer on the bench, the Supreme Court reversed its decision in *Commonwealth v. Gardner* and read an exemption into Sections 272 and 12 of the state penal code. Lewis Corbett, a pharmacist, had been found guilty in the superior court of violating the statutes in question for selling condoms. Corbett appealed his case to the state supreme court. Two years earlier, the Supreme Court had argued that it was not the job of the judicial branch of government to determine public policy. Now, however, Justice J. Lummus argued that, although it was clear that "the public policy of the Commonwealth . . . is offended by the sale of articles intended to prevent conception, . . . it does not appear to be any part of the public policy . . . to permit venereal disease to spread unchecked even among those who indulge in illicit sexual intercourse."[117] Thus, Lummus argued that it could not be proven that the defendant knew the condoms were to be used for illegal purposes, but, rather, was aware that they may well have been used in an effort to check the spread of disease. Lummus' interpretation of the statutes in question allowed for ambiguity and raised the question of intent to the degree that it would be difficult to prosecute sellers and disseminators of birth control in the Commonwealth. He completely reversed the earlier decision when he stated that "If our analysis of the language of the statute before us shows it to be less stringent than is desired, the remedy must be sought in the Legislature."[118] Thus, the Corbett decision put the burden of legislative reform on the shoulders of opponents of contraception rather than supporters. With this decision, the situation in Massachusetts began to resemble that of other states. Five years later, the Mothers' Health Council became part of the national planned parenthood movement, renaming itself for the last time the Planned Parenthood League of Massachusetts.

After resigning the presidency of the League, Ames continued to work for the legalization of birth control and for her holistic vision of reproductive reform. From the late 1940s through the early 1950s, Ames became a central figure in the controversy surrounding the fate of the New England Hospital for Women and Children (NEH). This hospital, created in 1863 to train women physicians and offer patients the opportunity to be treated by women, had fallen upon hard times by the 1940s. According to one historian, the hospital was "feminist in its conception and practice [and] flourished as the women's movement progressed."[119] As revenues fell, however, hospital administrators and funders recommended that men be added to hospital staff. The objective was ostensibly to help the hospital make a "transition from a special institution to a general community hospital staffed by men and women."[120]

As a member of the hospital's board of directors, Ames was one among a vocal minority that opposed the hiring of male doctors. She sought to continue the tradition of this unique women's health care institution, and worried that opening doors to male doctors would necessarily close some doors to women physicians. Challenges to the NEH continued and, in 1953, a report on improving hospital services recommended a merger with another area hospital. Ames interpreted this recommendation as another threat to the sanctity of this institution. At seventy-five years of age, she succeeded in staving off the merger and was elected president of the board of directors in the process.

Ames's dedication to preserving the NEH underscores the temerity of her reform spirit. By the 1950s, she was a seasoned veteran of battles in Massachusetts's politics. While women's suffrage and the legalization of birth control suffered from peculiarly vehement opposition in her home state, Ames had lived to see the success of both movements. Furthermore, her dedication to preserving the hospital illustrates the centrality of her commitment to women's health. As the NEH was acclaimed for its obstetrical and pediatric units, Ames's interest in its survival followed in the footsteps of her pioneering, if frustrating, work in the birth control movement. Although ostensibly a reproductive rights activist, her political career revolved around a commitment to reproductive health as well.

⊙⫯⊙

Ames's activities in the BCLM provide an example of the variety of ways birth control reformers attempted to frame their cause during the interwar years. A feminist and a pragmatist, Ames had to accommodate her league to the prevailing political climate in order to keep her movement viable. Distinguishing her state campaign from Sanger's and Dennett's national efforts, Ames struggled (not always successfully) to design a sustainable and suitable movement for Massachusetts. The overarching themes of the Massachusetts birth control movement—political pragmatism, deference to physicians, and the lack of success associated with these two carefully designed strategies—provides an interesting context for understanding Sanger's and Dennett's achievements, choices, and failures. For example, Sanger's shift toward a doctors-only strategy can be judged differently when compared to the BCLM's failures. In fact, the history of the BCLM shows that Sanger's efforts to negotiate the tricky terrain of coalition politics with physicians were ultimately rather savvy and successful, as Sanger never abdicated authority to the medical professionals to the same degree Ames did as president of the BCLM. The fate of the BCLM also sheds light on Dennett's clean repeal strategy. In light of the obstacles the League faced, we can see both the potential benefits as well as the unrealistic nature of Dennett's vision. While Dennett's strategies sought to evade the messiness and unpredictability of judicial interpretation, they required a legislative campaign and level of public acceptance of birth control that could not be counted on.

The case of the state league illustrates the various ways that reproductive reformers reacted to an unfriendly political climate with varying degrees of success. It also shows how different interpretations of the significance of birth control led reformers to publicize and strategize differently, creating alliances and associations that would greatly influence the shape and style of their movement. The BCLM's immediate postwar change to the Family Welfare Foundation represented a significant, but virtually ignored, political strategy among birth control reformers in the interwar years, as the league struggled to define its cause as an issue of life and death for women and children. The FWF envisioned a comprehensive reproductive reform agenda that included birth control among other maternal and infant welfare issues. However, birth control was never accepted among mainstream maternal and child welfare reformers, despite aggressive efforts on the part of some birth control reformers to completely revamp their rhetoric and strategies. Once birth control reformers in Massachusetts realized that neither other reproductive reformers nor the general public accepted this characterization of themselves, they moved, like Sanger, to advance their cause through the power of the organized medical community. Ames's career has shown that these decisions and shifts represented thoughtful political strategies as much as ideological reformulations of the issue.

Despite her constant strategical maneuvering, in an important sense, Ames's position remained fixed over the years; that is, she maintained a consistent commitment to the health and well-being of mothers and babies. Although political and legal circumstances would impel the use of varied tactics over the years—associating with maternalist causes, avoiding legislative activity on first the federal and then eventually the state level, asking for the leadership of physicians, relying on favorable court decisions, and opening medically supervised clinics—Ames began and ended her career in the birth control movement with a plea for the protection of women's lives. The trajectory of her activism, in its mutability and cohesion, illustrates the integral connection between issues of reproductive health and reproductive rights.

Epilogue

According to Kathryn Kish Sklar, "Women's political culture was not a natural outcome of . . . gender identity, but a consequence of particular social, political, and economic structures and values."[1] This study has sought to reveal and compare these particulars through the careers of four middle-class and elite white women who worked to aid mothers in the early decades of the twentieth century. Their careers help to explain how general concerns over motherhood and infancy became situated specifically in the political sphere in the pre- and postsuffrage eras, and how individual activists configured reproductive health and rights during a time of contested conceptions of reproduction, female sexuality, motherhood, public hygiene, and state responsibility.

Each woman in this study was part of a larger reproductive reform impulse that captured the energy of a wide variety of activists in the interwar years. However, their efforts never congealed into a comprehensive social welfare program to ameliorate the harsh conditions surrounding maternity and infancy. I have tried to show that this circumstance was neither inevitable, nor unproblematic. Clearly, there were individual reproductive reformers who envisioned a movement that would address the myriad concerns of mothers—including prenatal care, clean milk, financial security, and fertility control. However, political circumstances, both within the female reform community and externally, tended to obviate the realization of such goals.

The development of a unified political agenda and movement was undermined by a complex political climate in these decades. As this study has shown, individual women reformers not only held different ideas on the problems mothers faced and what needed to be done to solve these problems, but also on the strategies that should be employed. While women in the Children's Bureau who struggled for Sheppard-Towner were dedicated to education and a social-scientific approach to reproductive health, others felt sure that all the visiting nurses, free pamphlets, and baby shows in the world could not get to the root of the problem, which was woman's lack of control over her fertility. For birth controllers like Ames, unbridled childbearing was at the root of women's physical, economic, and civic debasement. Dennett would argue, more specifically, that the machinery of a repressive state apparatus hindered women in their ability to fully care for themselves and their families. Still others, like Putnam, argued that only improvements in and access to medical care— preferably accomplished on a private basis—could begin to put a dent in the high maternal and infant mortality rates. For her part, Dummer focused on the importance of economic justice and a revised moral and legal code in the fight for women's health and welfare. Despite the Children's Bureau's claim to have designed a holistic child welfare agenda, it omitted, overlooked, and/or rejected several strategies to aid the mothers of these children.

The agenda of the Bureau in the interwar years comes into sharper focus once we know of the existence of Ethel Dummer, who asked her friend Julia Lathrop if she would publicly support a progressive, European-inspired illegitimacy law. Alternately, she wondered if this was "too radical a stance" for someone in the Bureau to take? Dummer reminds us of roads not taken by the women who created a female dominion in child welfare, accentuating the differences between a child-centered and a woman-centered agenda. And studying one-time Bureau supporter Elizabeth Putnam, who liked to say of it, "the more statistics they pile up, the more we can see how absolutely nothing they have done," highlights the aggressiveness with which critics attacked the Bureau in the postwar period and makes the Bureau's proclivity toward compromise appear more sensible. Putnam's elitism also contextualizes the class politics of the Bureau, pointing to its sensitivity to the vulnerable and needy and its innovative approach to public health.

Similarly, the Sanger-led birth control movement takes on a new cast when examined from vantage points other than Sanger's. The careers of Dennett and Ames illustrate the difficulties of formulating an effective approach to securing reproductive rights. Dennett's attempt to claim for birth control the status of a "Constitutionally guaranteed old-fashioned American liberty" fell upon deaf ears on Capitol Hill. Rejecting the tradition and rhetoric of maternalism and formally lobbying for legislative reform, Dennett presaged the difficulties women would face once they moved into the formal political sphere. In contrast, Ames was thwarted in similar ways in her attempts to promote a decidedly modern reform agenda as part of a larger maternalist effort on behalf of mothers and children. Ames stood firm in her belief that birth control needed to become an integral part of the health care delivery system and classed it with other maternal health initiatives, despite continued rejection by policy makers. Together, the political challenges these activists faced serve to illustrate that, while the heyday of maternalism may have waned by the interwar years, another effective strategy had yet to emerge to take its place.

Debates among women reformers dedicated to reproductive health and rights need to be understood in their proper political context. Analyzing rhetoric and discourse about motherhood or sexuality may unveil assumptions regarding the shifting perceptions of womanhood, but widening one's gaze to examine political strategies and tactics reveals the ways in which women's reform culture intersected with the arenas of partisan or formal politics. My examination of individual political activists convinces me that what separated women reformers from one another in this period was more than their ideological positions on the proper role of women, the differences between men and women, and the nature of the nuclear family. Political affiliations and circumstances were as important in explaining their views on reproductive reform as was the level of their commitment to women's equality.

The failure to develop a comprehensive reproductive reform agenda has left a significant legacy on American society. Mothers and children still make up the overwhelming majority of those living in poverty, infant mortality is on the rise, antiabortion forces have moved from the margins to the center of power in the Republican Party, adolescent mothers have lost their rights to live independently and still be supported by the state, and, more generally, federal entitlements have lost credibility with a majority of the American public. The health *and* the rights of mothers and children are threatened by this constellation of cultural and political trends and policy decisions. Clearly, however, these trends cannot be blamed on reformers of the past. As this study has shown, even great insights and political astuteness have led nowhere in U.S. politics and policy. Although internal problems such as egos, temperaments, misjudgements, and insensitivities clearly existed, external obstacles are just as, if not more, significant in explaining the inability to develop and sustain a movement dedicated to a broad agenda of reproductive rights and health. Above all, popular resistance to changes in family structure, to programs that would increase women's autonomy and power and undermine the traditional family, kept reproductive reformers divided and on the defensive. In the face of such hostility, reformers carefully chose strategies designed to protect and promote defensive and, therefore, weakened agendas. These choices evolved out of deeply held personal beliefs as well as political considerations.

Throughout this study I have sought to round out our knowledge of the white women who shaped public policy and public attitudes in the arena of reproductive health and rights by examining the Sanger-dominated birth control movement and the policies emanating from the Children's Bureau's in the context of dialogue and dissent. Whether looking at outspoken rivalries, as in the cases of Putnam and Dennett, or the gentle prodding of constructive critics, like Dummer and Ames, we get insight into the political culture of white women in the decades after suffrage. These portraits provide a new perspective on the leaders of the reproductive rights and reproductive health movements in this country. They were not only battling bravely for the welfare of women and children, but striving to maintain their authority and to assert their vision in a complex and lively political climate rife with debate and dissent.

Reformers offered a variety of solutions to "the whole problem of motherhood" (in the words of Ethel Dummer) because they interpreted the problems of motherhood in different ways. The simple, yet profound, question that animated them still needs answering today: What can be done to help mothers? Answers ranged (and still range) from offers of solace and exhortations to behave responsibly to demands for social justice and equality. In between these two poles were campaigns to protect women's health, promote women's power, enhance the image of motherhood, get mothers more money and more control over their money, and alter family structure both culturally and legally. It is important to be mindful of the creativity, vitality, and variability of past efforts to improve the lives of mothers and children in light of the fact that these two groups have become the poorest, most vulnerable citizens not only in this country, but around the world.

Notes

Notes to Introduction

1. Dummer to Anthony, June 12, 1917, box 26, Ethel Sturges Dummer Papers (hereafter cited as ESD Papers).

2. Lynne Curry, *Modern Mothers in the Heartland* (Columbus: Ohio State University Press, 1999). For a brief, but comprehensive overview of women's voluntary activism around issues of social welfare see Paula Baker, "The Domestication of Politics: Women and American Political Society, 1780–1920," *American Historical Review* 89 (June 1984): 620–47. See also Carroll Smith-Rosenberg, *Disorderly Conduct: Visions of Gender in Victorian America* (New York: Oxford University Press, 1985); Barbara Leslie Epstein, *The Politics of Domesticity: Women, Evangelism, and Temperance in Nineteenth-Century America* (Middletown, Conn.: Wesleyan University Press, 1981); Ruth Bordin, *Women and Temperance: The Quest for Power and Liberty, 1873–1900* (Philadelphia: University of Pennsylvania Press, 1981); Karen J. Blair, *The Clubwoman as Feminist: True Womanhood Redefined, 1868–1914* (New York: Holmes & Meier Publishers, 1980); Mary P. Ryan, *Women in Public: From Banners to Ballots* (Baltimore, Md.: Johns Hopkins University Press, 1990).

3. Lynne Curry puts it another way when she writes that during the early twentieth century, "A broad coalition of public health practitioners, social welfare advocates, and women's rights supporters argued that a sound and democratic future depended upon mothers' ability to produce and maintain a robust citizenry." Curry, *Modern Mothers in the Heartland*, 1.

4. The exception to this is Carol R. McCann's *Birth Control Politics in the U.S., 1916–45* (Ithaca, N.Y.: Cornell University Press, 1994), which argues that birth control reformers need to be examined in the context of other reformers from the period, including "welfare feminists." She focuses on shared discourses such as the economic ethic of fertility, racial betterment, and racial liberalism.

5. Richard Meckel, *Save the Babies: American Public Health Reform and the Prevention of Infant Mortality, 1850–1929* (Baltimore, Md.: Johns Hopkins University Press, 1990), 5. According to Meckel, "the American discourse on infant mortality was

conducted as part of a somewhat larger discourse on national deterioration, depopulation and race suicide" (116).

6. Kriste Lindenmeyer, *"A Right to Childhood": The U.S. Children's Bureau and Child Welfare, 1912–46* (Urbana: University of Illinois Press, 1997), 19.

7. *Congressional Record*, 60th Cong., 2d sess., 1909, 43, 2897–98; quoted in Lindenmeyer, *"A Right to Childhood,"* 22.

8. Robyn Muncy, *Creating a Female Dominion in American Reform, 1890–1935* (New York: Oxford University Press, 1991), xii.

9. Meckel, *Save the Babies*, 5.

10. According to Sonya Michel, what separated maternalists from feminists in this era were the former's affirmation and the latter's rejection of the social structures that imposed dependency upon women. This distinction will become quite clear in chapter 2, when Dummer's feminism is counterpoised to both conservative and progressive maternalism.

11. Ladd-Taylor has focused on different ideas about gender roles to distinguish sentimental maternalists from progressive ones. My emphasis, however, is on the political environment within which women reformers operated. Therefore, I call Putnam a conservative maternalist, rather than a sentimental one, to underscore her ties with larger conservative political forces in the interwar years.

12. Indeed, there is certainly a link between the fact of Dummer's radicalism and her lack of political success, as chapter 2 will show. This link has been noted by historians studying women's political culture and maternalist activism. For example, according to Koven and Michel, in their edited volume on maternalist politics and the welfare state, "the fact that most of the women and movements we explore ultimately lacked the political power to refashion the state according to their own vision does not diminish the importance of that vision, their accomplishments, or their legacy." *Mothers of a New World: Maternalist Politics and the Origins of Welfare States* (New York: Routledge, 1993), 3. This interest in and respect for the politics of women "who dared to imagine what it would be like to enter into their newly born 'mother world,'" has inspired my own work on second-tier leaders.

Notes to Chapter 1

1. Elizabeth Putnam to Dr. Tagliaferro Clark, May 6, 1927, box 30, Elizabeth Lowell Putnam Papers (hereafter cited as ELP Papers).

2. Elizabeth Putnam to A. Piatt Andrew, March 8, 1929, box 16, ELP Papers. Although Coolidge gave lukewarm endorsement to the expansion of Sheppard-Towner in 1927, he made clear his desire to shift the responsibility for maternal and infant welfare from the federal government to the states. See Stanley J. Lemons, *The Woman Citizen: Social Feminism in the 1920s* (Urbana: University of Illinois Press, 1975), 173, 174.

3. Ladd-Taylor would categorize Putnam as a sentimental maternalist because of her conservative and specifically antisuffrage politics, but her ideas often clashed with the group represented in *Mother-Work* by the National Congress of Mothers as much as it did with feminists and progressive maternalists.

4. Koven and Michel, "Introduction: Mother Worlds," in *Mothers of a New World*, 4.

5. Putnam, "Woman and the Ballot," *Boston Common* (August 20, 1910) in ELP box 27, scrapbook volume 1, 128.

6. The first phrase is borrowed from Kathryn Kish Sklar. The quote comes from Koven and Michel, "Introduction: Mother Worlds," *Mothers of a New World*, 2.

7. While ideologically closest to the reformers Ladd-Taylor has called "sentimental maternalists," Putnam's politics cannot be captured by this description. Unlike these women who held staunchly to traditional notions of family and gender roles, and supported temperance and child labor reform, Putnam launched an impressive political career after the Nineteenth Amendment was passed. She also fought against prohibition and child labor reform, and even toyed with the idea of supporting birth control. Some of these seemingly odd or disparate positions stemmed from the realities of partisan politics; her choices became constrained as she rose in the ranks of the conservative wing of the Republican Party. Thus, her career suggests the need to expand our analysis of women's reform behavior into the larger context of political culture.

8. Linda Gordon, "Social Insurance and Public Assistance: The Influence of Gender in Welfare Thought in the United States, 1890–1935," *American Historical Review* 97 (February 1992): 19–54. In addition, see Virginia Sapiro, Barbara Nelson, and Gwendolyn Mink. The CB certainly had its flaws when it came to the policies it developed on behalf of women and children (especially the former), as has been well documented by the above-mentioned historians as well as, more recently, by Sonya Michel in her groundbreaking book *Children's Interests/Mothers' Rights* (New Haven, Conn.: Yale University Press, 1999). The Bureau's shortcomings will be made abundantly clear in the next chapter. However, for the purposes of putting the work of individual reformers into context (one of the fundamental aims of this project), Putnam's activities on behalf of mothers and infants are as important as the activities of those feminists whose work we have admired. I argue that activists like Putnam, who made absolutely no attempt to cross class, ethnic, or racial boundaries, mitigate the CB's awkwardness in these areas.

9. "Hoover Cold to Boston Move to Abolish Children's Bureau," *The Sun*, March 4, 1930.

10. Meckel, *Save the Babies*, 62.

11. Ibid., 68.

12. Ibid., 69.

13. Massachusetts Milk Consumers Association bulletin, n.d., box 8, ELP Papers.

14. Putnam to editor of the *Worcester Telegram*, October 6, 1911, box 4, ELP Papers.

15. Ibid.

16. Barbara Gutmann Rosenkrantz, *Public Health and the State: Changing Views in Massachusetts, 1842–1936* (Cambridge, Mass.: Harvard University Press, 1972), 135.

17. Ibid., 107.

18. Ibid., 108.

19. Ibid., 109.

20. Putnam to William Taft, August 14, 1909, box 6, ELP Papers.

21. Putnam's preference for a clean milk supply was echoed by the leaders in the public health arena in her home state. The monthly *Bulletin for the State Board of Health* in 1906 argued against an overreliance on "municipal milk stations and philanthropic distribution" and for clean milk and breast-feeding.

22. Kathryn Kish Sklar, "'Brain Work for Women'": Women, Social Science, and the American Welfare State in the Progressive Era." Paper presented at the Eighth Berkshire Conference in Women's History, Douglass College, New Brunswick, N.J., June 1990.

23. *Women's Municipal League Bulletin,* 1912, box 4, ELP Papers.

24. Putnam to Mrs. Mulligan, January 23, 1912, box 7, ELP Papers.

25. Putnam "Suggestions on Prenatal Care Founded on a Five Year Experiment," read before AASPIM, November 1914, box 4, ELP Papers.

26. In 1915, neonatal mortality rates (deaths within the first month) were 4.3 percent, according to the National Center for Health Statistics. Meckel, *Save the Babies,* 239.

27. Ibid.

28. Putnam, final draft of article for *Modern Hospital,* November 2, 1917, box 3, ELP Papers. This article was published in the February 1918 issue of the *Modern Hospital.* It is noted that the published article contains part of the report made by Elizabeth Lowell Putnam to the AASPIM, box 28, ELP Papers.

29. Ibid.

30. Richard W. Wertz and Dorothy C. Wertz, *Lying In: A History of Childbirth in America* (New York: Schocken, 1979), 136–38.

31. See Robyn Muncy, *Creating a Female Dominion in American Reform;* Linda Gordon, *Pitied but Not Entitled: Single Mothers and the History of Welfare, 1890–1935* (New York: Free Press, 1994); Kriste Lindenmeyer, *"A Right to Childhood";* Gwendolyn Mink, *Wages of Motherhood: Inequality in the Welfare State, 1917–1942* (Ithaca, N.Y.: Cornell University Press, 1995); and Sonya Michel, *Children's Interests/Mother's Rights.*

32. Putnam, final draft of article for *Modern Hospital,* November 2, 1917.

33. Putnam, "Prenatal Care of the Next Generation," *Survey,* January 4, 1913, box 3, ELP Papers.

34. Muncy, *Creating a Female Dominion in American Reform,* 143.

35. Putnam, untitled address, n.d., box 3, ELP Papers.

36. Putnam, *Women's Municipal League Bulletin,* 1912, box 4, ELP Papers.

37. Meckel, *Save the Babies,* 109.

38. Senate Bill no. 506, enclosed in a letter from Massachusetts Congressman B. L. Young, Committee on Rules to Putnam, April 26, 1920, box 16, ELP Papers.

39. B. L. Young to Putnam, April 26, 1920, box 16, ELP Papers.

40. Putnam to Frank G. Allen, May 12, 1920, box 16, ELP Papers.

41. Mrs. Max West to Putnam, November 25, 1912, box 30, ELP Papers.

42. Putnam to Mrs. Max West, March 17, 1913, box 30, ELP Papers.

43. Ibid.

44. Julia Lathrop to Putnam, October 31, 1912, box 9, ELP Papers.

45. Julia Lathrop to Putnam, November 14, 1912, box 30, ELP Papers.

46. Julia Lathrop to Putnam, November 5, 1912, box 30, ELP Papers.

47. Putnam to Julia Lathrop, November 12, 1912, box 30, ELP Papers.

48. The first milk station was established in New York City in 1892. Meckel, *Save the Babies,* 78.

49. Putnam to Senator Henry Cabot Lodge, April 10, 1914, box 30, ELP Papers. It was noted at the bottom of the letter that a copy was sent to representative Gardner and Senator Weeks. Florence Kelley and Julia Lathrop asked Lovejoy to initiate a letter-writing campaign on behalf of the CB once the House Committee on Appro-

priations denied the Bureau's request for increased funding. Lovejoy sent letters predominantly to NCLC members for signs of support. Putnam was no supporter of the NCLC; she opposed child labor reform as an unnecessary intrusion into the economy and family life. That Putnam received one and then went on to respond to his request illustrates the complexity of reproductive reform politics.

50. Putnam, Presidential Address to the AASPIM, December 1918, box 4, ELP Papers.

51. In 1916 Mrs. West, author of the Bureau's *Prenatal Care*, asked Putnam to send materials to the Health Officer from Liverpool, England, who requested practical information on setting up prenatal care programs. In 1918, Lathrop relied on Putnam to be host to a visiting dignitary from New Zealand who had done important work on maternal and infant welfare. West to Putnam, April 1, 1916, Children's Bureau-Central File (CB-CF) 4-15-4-1-1; Lathrop to Putnam, January 15, 1918, CB-CF 4-15-5-0-1.

52. Putnam to Dr. George Vincent, January 9, 1918, box 15, ELP Papers.

53. Lathrop to Putnam, February 9, 1918, CB-CF, File 9-4-1.

54. Jane Jerome, *Women Against Women* (Brooklyn, N.Y.: Carlson, 1994).

55. Putnam to editor of the *New York Post*, "Women and the Campaign," August 30, 1916, box 3, ELP Papers.

56. Ironically, Putnam's words can be seen as echoing the position of one of the key feminist theorists of the early twentieth century, Charlotte Perkins Gilman. Only one year earlier, in 1915, Gilman spoke of the "overwhelming mass of sentiment on the side of continuous indulgence" in relation to the birth control question. In the same article (*Forerunner* 6, no. 7 [July 1915]: 176) she also named "a desire for 'safe' and free indulgence of the sex instinct without this natural consequence" as one of the main reasons behind the birth control movement. Despite these critiques, Gilman gave her first half-hearted endorsement of birth control in this same issue of the magazine. Presaging the direction of the Sanger-led movement, Gilman argued that physicians should have the right to teach such practices to their patients at their discretion.

57. Putnam, presidential address to AASPIM, Dec 1918.

58. Ibid.

59. Charles Zeublin to Putnam, September 30, 1916, box 30, ELP Papers.

60. Charles Zeublin to Putnam, September 2, 1916, box 30, ELP Papers.

61. Ibid.

62. Putnam to BCLM, September 26, 1916, box 30, ELP Papers.

63. Mary East to Putnam, April 1917, box 30, ELP Papers.

64. Vera P. Lane to Putnam, August 4, 1919, box 30, ELP Papers.

65. Mary Ware Dennett to Putnam, September 9, 1919, box 30, ELP Papers.

66. Putnam to Senator Henry Cabot Lodge, January 5, 1921, box 17, ELP Papers.

67. Louis J. Covotsos, "Child Welfare and Social Progress: A History of the United States Children's Bureau, 1912–35" (Ph.D. diss., University of Chicago, 1976).

68. Dr. S. Josephine Baker, address before Committee on Labor of the House of Representatives, Washington, D.C., January 28, 1919, box 16, ELP Papers.

69. Putnam to Henry Cabot Lodge, May 17, 1921, box 17, ELP Papers.

70. Ibid.

71. Ibid.

72. Anon., "Reasons Why the Administration of the Sheppard-Towner Bill Should Be Vested in the Children's Bureau," n.d., box 1, Dorothy Kirchwey Brown Papers (hereafter cited as DKB Papers).

73. Putnam, address, n.d., box 3, ELP Papers. To a certain extent, Putnam's comment reflected a valid critique of the purely educational focus of Sheppard-Towner— one that may have come from the right or the left.

74. Putnam, "The Sheppard-Towner Bill," *JAMA* 76 (April 30, 1921): 1264–65; Dorothy Kirchwey Brown to editor, *JAMA,* March 9, 1922, box 1, DKB Papers.

75. Putnam to Charles Powles, March 16, 1916; Putnam to Dr. George Kosmak, February 7, 1919, box 16, ELP Papers.

76. Putnam to Henry Cabot Lodge, May 17, 1921, box 17, ELP Papers.

77. Putnam to Col. Winslow, December 14, 1921, box 17, ELP Papers.

78. Putnam, letter to *JAMA,* 1921, box 3, ELP Papers.

79. See for example, Putnam, speech before the Tuesday Club, December 1, 1925, box 29, scrapbook, ELP Papers.

80. Putnam to the editor of the *Springfield Republican,* February 10, 1924, box 16, ELP Papers.

81. Williams, "The Midwife Problem," quoted in Meckel, *Save the Babies,* 174.

82. Lindenmeyer, *"A Right to Childhood,"* 96.

83. Muncy, *Creating a Female Dominion in American Reform,* 116.

84. Putnam to the editor of the *Independent,* January 6, 1926, box 30, ELP Papers. The first part of quote also came from Putnam's speech before the Tuesday Club, Cambridge, Mass., December 1, 1925, box 29, ELP Papers.

85. Putnam to William Graham, February 19, 1926, box 30, ELP Papers.

86. Putnam to A. Piatt Andrew, January 31, 1929, box 16, ELP Papers.

87. Putnam to Dr. George Kosmak, January 31, 1929, box 16, ELP Papers.

88. Putnam, speech before Daughters of 1812, March 1930, box 4, ELP Papers.

89. Putnam, "Increased Federalization," n.d. (probably 1929–31) box 4, 57, ELP Papers.

90. Putnam, speech before Daughters of 1812, March 1930, box 4, 48, ELP Papers.

91. Putnam, notes on Grace Abbott, January 18, 1931, box 16, ELP Papers (Italics mine).

92. Putnam, "Establishment of the Children's Bureau," n.d., box 17, ELP Papers.

93. Ibid.

94. Lynn Dumenil, "'The Insatiable Maw of Bureaucracy': Antistatism and Education Reform in the 1920s," *Journal of American History* 77 (September 1990): 499–524.

95. Putnam to A. Piatt Andrew, March 8, 1929, box 16, ELP Papers.

96. Putnam to Dr. Tagliaferro Clark, May 6, 1927, box 30, 511, ELP Papers.

97. Putnam to A. Piatt Andrew, March 8, 1929, box 16, ELP Papers

98. Putnam to Dr. Tagliaferro Clark, October 26, 1929, box 16, ELP Papers.

99. Ibid.

100. Putnam to Dr. Kosmak, February 7, 1929, box 16, ELP Papers.

101. Putnam to Dr. Tagliaferro Clark, October 26, 1929, box 16, ELP Papers.

102. Ibid.

103. Putnam to A. Piatt Andrew, February 27, 1930, box 16, ELP Papers.

104. Huthmacher, *Massachusetts People and Politics, 1919–1933* (New York: Atheneum, 1969), 69–71. Huthmacher's quote from Cardinal O'Connell spells out

these dynamics: "The medical inspection of schools, the physical examination and treatment of school children, the supplying of food for the indigent pupil, free dispensary treatment for the defective, and other similar provisions which have all been added to the education program of the state, all are signs of the spirit of machine centralization and control . . . which should be abandoned," 69.

105. "Who Controls our Children," *Boston Traveler,* March 5, 1930, box 29, scrapbook, ELP Papers.

106. *Boston Herald,* March 12, 1930.

107. Putnam to Robert L. Dickinson, January 21, 1927, box 30, ELP Papers.

108. Putnam, speech before the Parliamentary Law Club, April 5, 1927, box 29, scrapbook, ELP Papers.

109. Putnam's attempt to add levity to her speech went even further when she offered an example of an offensive limerick that should not be censored, "first, because although portraying vice, it makes evil thoroughly unattractive; and second, because I do not want my grandchildren singing it around the street, as they doubtless would were it censored." Putnam, speech, April 5, 1927.

110. Putnam to Mrs. Ada Price, president of the Florida branch of the Coolidge Women's Club of America, October 29, 1930, box 25, ELP Papers.

111. Putnam to Slattery, June 20, 1930, box 16, 297, ELP Papers.

112. Kathryn Kish Sklar, "'Brain Work for Women.'"

Notes to Chapter 2

1. Dummer, "Some Thoughts on Life and Love," 1920, box 16, ESD Papers.

2. Anthony Platt, *The Child Savers: The Invention of Delinquency* (Chicago: University of Chicago Press, 1969), 24, 25.

3. Dummer to W. I. Thomas, June 9, 1921, box 36, folder 785, ESD Papers, quoted in Platt, "Acting as a Switchboard," 25.

4. Wendy Sarvasy, "Beyond the Difference versus Equality Policy Debate: Postsuffrage Feminism, Citizenship, and the Quest for a Feminist Welfare State," *Signs* 17 (winter 1992): 332.

5. On the notion that infant and maternal death acted as a catalyst for the politicization of motherhood, see Molly Ladd-Taylor, *Mother-Work: Women, Child Welfare, and the State, 1890–1930* (Urbana: University of Illinois Press, 1994), 18–20.

6. Ethel Sturges Dummer, *Why I Think So: The Autobiography an Hypothesis* (Chicago: Clarke-McElroy Publishing Co., 1937), 33.

7. Ibid., 33.

8. Ibid., 35.

9. Ibid., 40.

10. On the significance of the University of Chicago in the development of the social sciences in the Progressive Era, see Ellen Fitzpatrick, *Endless Crusade: Women Social Scientists and Progressive Reform* (New York: Oxford University Press, 1990); Mary Jo Deegan, *Jane Addams and the Men of the Chicago School, 1892–1918* (New Brunswick, N.J.: Transaction Books, 1990, c1988); Allen F. Davis, *Spearheads for Reform: The Social Settlements and the Progressive Movement, 1890–1914* (New Brunswick, N.J.: Rutgers University Press, 1984); Thomas Haskell, *The Emergence of Professional Social Science* (Urbana: University of Illinois Press, 1977); Lawrence Veysey,

Emergence of the American University (Chicago: University of Chicago Press, 1965); Margaret W. Rossiter, *Woman Scientists in America* (Baltimore, Md.: Johns Hopkins University Press, 1982), ch. 1 and 2.

11. Muncy, *Creating a Female Dominion in American Reform*, 66.

12. Mary Odem, *Delinquent Daughters: Protecting and Policing Adolescent Female Sexuality in the United States, 1885–1920* (Chapel Hill: University of North Carolina Press, 1995), 111.

13. Healy went on to an auspicious career, becoming Director of the Juvenile Psychopathic Institute, publishing several studies of delinquency, and directing the Judge Baker Foundation in Boston. Named after a leader in the juvenile court movement, the Baker Foundation sought to investigate the variable causal factors involved in delinquent behavior. On Judge Baker's contributions to the juvenile justice system and the Foundation named after him, see William Healy, *Harvey Humphrey Baker: Upbuilder of the Juvenile Court* (Boston: Judge Baker Foundation Publications, 1920). Examples of Healy's more empirical and fairminded investigations of delinquents are *The Individual Delinquent* (Boston: Little, Brown, 1915) and *Delinquents and Criminals* (co-authored with Augusta F. Bronner; New York: MacMillan, 1926). Jennifer Platt suggests that Dummer played a vital role in Healy's "very consequential appointment" to the Psychopathic Institute in "Acting as a Switchboard."

14. Odem, *Delinquent Daughters*, 156. For more on the juvenile courts, see also David Rothman, *Conscience and Convenience: The Asylum and Its Alternatives in Progressive America* (Boston: Little, Brown, 1980); Steven L. Schlossman, *Love and the American Delinquent: The Theory and Practice of "Progressive" Juvenile Justice* (Chicago, University of Chicago Press, 1970); Eric C. Schneider, *In the Web of Class: Delinquents and Reformers in Boston, 1810s–1930s* (New York: New York University Press, 1992); Ellen Ryerson, *Best Laid Plans: America's Juvenile Court Experiment* (New York: Hill & Wang, 1978); Anthony Platt, *The Child Savers*; Susan Tiffin, *In Whose Best Interest? Child Welfare Reform in the Progressive Era* (Westport, Conn.: Greenwood Press, 1982).

15. Estelle Freedman writes in her biography of penologist Miriam Van Waters that 25 percent of the girls brought to the Los Angeles Juvenile Hall were pregnant.

16. See Linda Gordon, "Black and White Visions of Welfare: Women's Welfare Activism, 1890–1945," *Journal of American History* 78 (September 1991): 559–90; and Susan Tiffin, *In Whose Best Interest?*. Kunzel argues in *Fallen Women* that social workers began by the 1920s to encourage white women to give up their illegitimate children for adoption, arguing that they were unfit mothers, whereas earlier evangelical reformers had faith in "the redemptive power of motherhood." Regina K. Kunzel, *Fallen Women, Problem Girls: Unmarried Mothers and the Professionalization of Social Work, 1890–1945* (New Haven, Conn.: Yale University Press, 1993). Although I agree that the latter position implied a potentially radical acceptance of single-parent families as legitimate families, my research has shown that the position could come out of a feminist as well as an evangelical orientation.

17. Dummer, *Why I Think So*, 54.

18. Ellen Key enjoyed much more notariety in the United States than Stöcker due to the publication of her books *The Century of the Child* (New York: Putnam, 1909) and *The Renaissance of Motherhood* (New York, 1914).

19. On Helene Stöcker and the BfM see Ann Taylor Allen, *Feminism and Motherhood in Germany, 1800–1914* (New Brunswick, N.J.: Rutgers University Press, 1991); Ann Taylor Allen, "Mothers of the New Generation Adele Schreiber, Helene

Stoecker, and the Evolution of a German Idea of Motherhood," *Signs* 10 (spring 1985): 418–38; Amy Hacket, "Helene Stoecker: Left-Wing Intellectual and Sex Reformer," in *When Biology Became Destiny: Women in Weimar and Nazi Germany,* ed. Bridenthal et al., 109–30 (New York: Monthly Review Press, 1984.); Amy Hacket, "The Politics of Feminism in Wilhelmine Germany 1880–1918" (Ph.D. diss., Columbia University, 1976); Atina Grossman, "The New Woman, the New Family and the Rationalization of Sexuality in Weimar Germany," in *Powers of Desire: The Politics of Sexuality,* ed. Ann Snitow et al., 153–76 (New York: Monthly Review Press, 1983); Atina Grossman, *Reforming Sex: The German Movement for Birth Control and Abortion Reform, 1920–1950* (New York: Oxford University Press, 1995); and Katharine Anthony, *Feminism in Germany and Scandinavia* (New York: Henry Holt, 1915).

20. Grossmann, *Reforming Sex,* 49.

21. Dummer, *Why I Think So,* 60.

22. Ibid.

23. Dummer to Kellogg, n.d., box 16, ESD Papers.

24. See Mari Jo Buhle, *Women and American Socialism, 1870–1920* (Urbana: University of Illinois Press, 1981).

25. Ibid., 260.

26. This quote is from David Leigh's article, "Emma Goldman in San Francisco," *Mother Earth* 10, no. 8 (October 1915): 277.

27. Within the reproductive reform community, it was Sanger who would gain inspiration from this group of American radicals. Dummer avoided direct activism related to free love and birth control, although her ideas about *Mutterschutz* certainly encompassed both issues, albeit in a more romanticized form. Sanger also developed a relationship with Stöcker, although one in which Sanger exhibited much less deference to the German philosopher and activist than did Dummer. By the 1920s Stöcker counted Dummer and Sanger among her important American contacts and asked both women to sponsor a trip to the States. In 1925 Sanger helped Stöcker travel to the neo-Malthusian conference in New York.

28. Lathrop, letter of transmittal, *Norwegian Laws Concerning Illegitimate Children* (Washington, D.C.: Children's Bureau Publication, legal series no. 1, Bureau publication no. 31, 1918).

29. Estelle Freedman, *Maternal Justice: Miriam Van Waters and the Female Reform Tradition* (Chicago: University of Chicago Press, 1996), 190.

30. Ten years after *Feminism in Germany and Scandinavia* was published, Anthony was still in contact with Stöcker, trying to arrange funding for a lecture tour in America, and securing her a place on the program at the sixth International Neo-Malthusian and Birth Control Conference (New York, 1925).

31. Anthony also fits into this analysis of reproductive reformers because of her interest in birth control and her connection to the radical feminist group, Heterodoxy. Mary Dennett had ties to this Greenwich Village group as well.

32. Anthony, *Feminism in Germany and Scandinavia,* 10. Subsequent studies of the suffrage movements in the West have built on or confirmed Anthony's original insights and interpretations. On German feminism, see Allen, *Feminism and Motherhood.* On France's "relational," "familial," or "maternal" feminism in this period, see Karen Offen, "Depopulation, Nationalism, and Feminism in Fin-de-Siecle France," *American Historical Review* 89 (1984): 654; and "Defining Feminism: A Comparative Historical Approach," *Signs* 14 (1988): 119–57.

33. Anthony, *Feminism in Germany and Scandinavia*, 87, 88.

34. Dummer to Anthony, March 21, 1916, box 26, ESD Papers.

35. Ibid.

36. Anthony to Dummer, April, 10, 1916, box 26, ESD Papers.

37. Dummer to Julia Lathrop, March 13, 1917, box 32, ESD Papers.

38. Charlotte Perkins Gilman, "As to War-Brides," *The Forerunner* 6, no. 3 (March 1915): 62.

39. For a brief discussion of the ideological differences between Gilman and Key, see Nancy Cott, *The Grounding of Modern Feminism* (New Haven, Conn.: Yale University Press, 1987), 46–49.

40. Lucy Waite to Dummer, June 23, 1917, box 23, ESD Papers.

41. Dummer to Paul Kellogg, n.d., box 16, ESD Papers.

42. Tiffin, *In Whose Best Interest?*, 43.

43. Gordon, *Pitied but Not Entitled*, 29

44. Dummer to Lathrop, April 9, 1917, box 32, ESD Papers. (Also File 10,551 Children's Bureau Records, Central Files, 1914–1920, Records Group 102, National Archives, Washington, D.C.)

45. Ibid.

46. Dummer to Julia Lathrop, August 30, 1916, box 32, ESD Papers.

47. Dummer to Anthony, February 12, 1917, box 26, ESD Papers.

48. Ibid.

49. Ibid.

50. Fitzpatrick provides a good background on Freund's education and political orientation in *Endless Crusade*. She does not mention his work on illegitimacy, but places him squarely within the Progressive social science community in Chicago. Freund was one of Sophonisba Breckinridge's mentors at the University of Chicago.

51. Kunzel, *Fallen Women, Problem Girls;* Mary Jo Deegan, *Jane Addams and the Men of the Chicago School, 1892–1918;* Costin, *Two Sisters for Social Justice: A Biography of Grace and Edith Abbott* (Urbana: University of Illinois Press, 1983); Muncy, *Creating a Female Dominion in American Reform;* Fitzpatrick, *Endless Crusade.*

52. Emma O. Lundberg to Julia Lathrop, memorandum, September 29, 1916, File 7361.8, CB-CF.

53. Dummer to Julia Lathrop, March 13, 1917, box 32, ESD Papers.

54. Dummer to Freund, March 18, 1917, box 32, ESD Papers.

55. Dummer to Katharine Anthony, May 10, 1921, box 26, ESD Papers.

56. Covotsos, "Child Welfare and Social Progress," 226.

57. Barbara Nelson, "The Origins of the Two-Channel Welfare State: Workmen's Compensation and Mothers' Aid," in *Women, the State, and Welfare*, ed. Linda Gordon (Madison: University of Wisconsin Press, 1990), 133.

58. Dummer to Katharine Anthony, June 12, 1917, box 26, ESD Papers.

59. Ibid.

60. Fosdick was a lawyer and reformer who eventually became head of the U. S. Public Health Service.

61. Allan M. Brandt, *No Magic Bullet: A Social History of Venereal Disease in the United States Since 1880* (New York: Oxford University Press, 1987), 94.

62. Ibid., 82.

63. Odem, *Delinquent Daughters*, 126.

64. Dummer to Fosdick, September 27, 1917, box 24, ESD Papers.

65. Dummer to Katharine Anthony, August 14, 1918, box 26, ESD Papers.

66. Dummer to Lathrop, October 20, 1917, box 32, ESD Papers.

67. Dummer to Lathrop, September 25, 1917, box 32, ESD Papers.

68. Dummer to Lathrop, October 20, 1917, box 32, ESD Papers.

69. Dummer to Lathrop, quoted in Dummer, *Why I Think So*, 88.

70. Brandt, *No Magic Bullet*, 84. Hobson's *Uneasy Virtue* refers to "An Act to Extend Protection to the Civil Rights of Members of Military and Naval Establishments" (in a note, 255). Barbara Meil Hobson, *Uneasy Virtue: The Politics of Prostitution and the American Reform Tradition* (New York: Basic Books, 1987).

71. Dummer to Binford, December 24, 1918, box 25, ESD Papers.

72. Dummer to Rippen, July 1918, box 24, ESD Papers.

73. In the 1910s, effective drugs to treat tuberculosis had not been discovered. The only treatment involved boosting the patient's immune system through a regime of rest, exposure to fresh air, good food and sunlight. Penologist Miriam Van Waters, who would enjoy Dummer's patronage in the postwar period, also suffered from this affliction. See Freedman, *Maternal Justice*, 65.

74. Dummer to Binford, February 21, 1921, box 25, ESD Papers.

75. Ibid.

76. Binford to Dummer, Feb 9, 1920, box 25, ESD Papers.

77. Freund, "A Uniform Illegitimacy Law," *Survey*, October 15, 1922.

78. Ibid.

79. Ibid.

80. Lousie De Koven Bowen, "Birth Registration and Establishment of Paternity: Determination and Recording of Parentage," *Standards of Legal Protection for Children Born Out of Wedlock: A Report of Regional Conferences*, Bureau Publication no. 77 (Washington, D.C.: Government Printing Office, 1921), 58.

81. Lathrop, letter of transmittal, *Standards of Legal Protection for Children Born Out Of Wedlock*, 7.

82. Lundberg to Freund, September 27, 1921, File 10-13-0, CB-CF.

83. Tiffin, *In Whose Best Interest?*, 181, 182.

84. Emma O. Lundberg and Katherine Lenroot, *Illegitimacy as a Child Welfare Problem*, Children's Bureau Publication no. 66 (Washington, D.C.: Government Printing Office, 1920).

85. Ibid., 8.

86. See Tiffin, *In Whose Best Interest?*

87. For more on the Children's Bureau and its conservative position on mothers' pensions, see Sonya Michel, *Children's Interests/Mothers' Rights*, ch. 2 and 3.

88. Leff, "Consensus for Reform: The Mothers' Pension Movement in the Progressive Era," in *Compassion and Responsibility: Readings in the History of Social Welfare Policy in the United States*, ed. Frank R. Breul and Steven J. Diner (Chicago: University of Chicago Press, 1980), 244. See also Joanne Goodwin, *Gender and the Politics of Welfare Reform* (Chicago: University of Chicago Press, 1997).

89. Tiffin, *In Whose Best Interest?*, 110.

90. Dummer, notes on Anthony's contributions to *The Endowment of Motherhood*, November 9, 1920, box 24, ESD Papers.

91. Sarvasy, "Beyond the Difference versus Equality Policy Debate," 341.

92. Anthony, ed., *The Endowment of Motherhood*, xi. Anthony and Dummer's vision of welfare once again defied the conventions associated with their race and class.

According to Linda Gordon, white middle-class women reformers in the first decades of the twentieth century generally supported means-tested social programs, accepted the family wage, and viewed mothers' pensions as a way to restore marriages.

93. Dummer to Lathrop, July 1921, box 32, ESD Papers.

94. On the connections between social science and social reform and the gendered forms this linkage often took in the Progressive Era, see Ellen Fitzpatrick, *Endless Crusade;* Leila Costin, *Two Sisters For Social Justice;* Muncy, *Creating a Female Dominion in American Reform;* Sklar, "'Brain Work for Women.'"

95. Copy of official statement written by Dummer regarding the funding and purpose of Thomas's research for *The Unadjusted Girl,* box 36, ESD Papers.

96. Fitzpatrick, *Endless Crusade,* 56.

97. For biographical information on Van Waters, see Freedman, *Maternal Justice.*

98. Ibid., 90.

99. Miriam Van Waters, speech at Dummer's memorial, March 7, 1954, box 15, ESD Papers.

100. Freedman, *Maternal Justice,* 98.

101. Ibid.

102. Ibid.

103. Ibid., xiii.

104. My understanding of the feminist position on maternal endowment was enhanced by the brief discussion in Ladd-Taylor's *Mother-Work,* 112–21.

105. Dummer to Katharine Anthony, May 10, 1921, box 26, ESD Papers.

106. Freedman, *Maternal Justice,* 115.

107. Muncy, *Creating a Female Dominion in American Reform,* 85.

108. Dummer, notes on *Endowment,* November 9, 1920.

Notes to Chapter 3

1. For more information on Dennett's divorce and subsequent life as a single mother, see Constance M. Chen, *The Sex Side of Life: Mary Ware Dennett's Pioneering Battle for Birth Control and Sex Education* (New York: New York University Press, 1996).

2. Although Sanger subsequently accused her of political timidity, Dennett's associations and activities during the war put her on par with any of the radical company Sanger herself kept.

3. Although critical of Sanger in *WBWR,* Gordon tends to perpetuate Sanger's own dismissal of Dennett as a conservative, bourgeois reformer. Chesler perpetuates Gordon's harsh assessment of Dennett when she writes, "Paradoxically, the more conservative Dennett held out adamantly for the total repeal of obscenity statutes on free speech grounds." In the absence of clear understanding of the nature of Dennett's politics, this description does seem paradoxical. However, this study will explore the ideologies that made these positions logically consistent. Chen's biography of Dennett is helpful in clarifying certain facts, but fails to provide sufficient attention to context. While adept at evoking Dennett's personality traits and recording the major events of her life in a lively fashion, Chen does not move the discussion of Sanger and Dennett any further along. She tends to swing the pendulum in favor of Dennett's version of the story, offering neither a critique of Dennett's position nor an analysis of the rift between

the two women. Instead of analysis, Chen offers the following attacks on Sanger: "Like other unthinking people, whether liberal or conservative, Sanger was myopic and intolerant" (162) and "Unlike Sanger whose hysterical outbursts early in her career had alienated so many, Dennett was an experienced reformer." (183) Thus, she shifts the historiography from Sanger's assessment of Dennett to Dennett's assessment of Sanger without proper historical analysis of their rivalry, its ideological underpinnings, or its place within larger discussions about maternal health, welfare and rights.

4. There has been much written about the limits that the maternalist philosophy and strategy placed on the CB. See Molly Ladd-Taylor, Sonya Michel, Linda Gordon, Gwendolyn Mink, Carole McCann.

5. Sanger had announced the creation of the National Birth Control League in the *Woman Rebel* before her trip to Europe in 1915, during which time the League took shape under the direction and leadership of Dennett and her middle-class colleagues. Although within a few years Sanger would be directing her appeal to a fundamentally middle-and upper-class audience, including physicians and politicians, in 1915 she was still associated with birth control radicalism and the Left.

6. Sanger, *Margaret Sanger: An Autobiography* (New York: Dover Publications, 1971), 180.

7. See Gordon, *Woman's Body, Woman's Right;* Lemons, *The Woman Citizen;* Cott, "What's In a Name? The Limits of 'Social Feminism'; or, Expanding the Vocabulary of Women's History," *Journal of American History* 76 (December 1989): 809–29.

8. Gordon tends to do this in *WBWR*.

9. Mary Ware Dennett, *Birth Control Laws: Shall We Keep Them, Change Them, or Abolish Them?* (New York: Grafton Press, 1936), 67.

10. Ibid., 66.

11. Ibid., 167.

12. Ibid., 171.

13. Ibid., 170.

14. Ibid., 171.

15. In fact, both women moved to New York City in the same year. For more on Sanger's years in the city, see Ellen Chesler, *Woman of Valor: Margaret Sanger and the Birth Control Movement in America* (New York: Simon and Schuster, 1992), chs. 3, 4, and 5. For more on Dennett's political and personal experiences, see Chen, *The Sex Side of Life,* chs. 9–12.

16. Dennett to Estelle Stewart, December 14, 1916, box 37, Mary Ware Dennett Papers (hereafter cited as MWD Papers). Quoted in Chen, *The Sex Side of Life,* 353.

17. Dennett to Anna Howard Shaw, August 17, 1912, box 12, MWD Papers. Quoted in Chen, *The Sex Side of Life,* 142.

18. On the Woman's Peace Party and women's peace activism more generally, see Harriet Alonso, *The Women's Peace Union and the Outlawry of War, 1921–1942* (Knoxville: University of Tennessee Press, 1989); Marie Louise Degen, *The History of the Woman's Peace Party* (Baltimore, Md.: Johns Hopkins University Press, 1939); John C. Farrell, *Beloved Lady: A History of Jane Addams' Ideas on Peace and Reform* (Baltimore, Md.: Johns Hopkins University Press, 1967); Blanche Cook ed., *Crystal Eastman on Women and Revolution* (New York: Oxford, 1979); Joan Jensen, "All Pink Sisters: The War Department and the Feminist Movement in the 1920s," in *Decades of Discontent: The Women's Movement 1920–1940,* ed. Lois Scharf and Joan Jensen (Boston: Northeastern University Press, 1987), 199–222.

19. For an explanation of the ideological connections between feminism, peace, and civil liberties, see Frances H. Early, "Feminism, Peace, and Civil Liberties: Women's Role in the Origins of the World War One Civil Liberties Movement," *Women's Studies* 18 (1990): 95–115.

20. "Doctors-only" legislation refers to Sanger's strategy from 1918 on to fight for the exemption of physicians from prohibitions against the distribution of contraceptives. This type of law would leave contraceptives under the rubric of obscenity as defined by the federal Comstock Laws, and not protect laypeople from prosecution.

21. Dennett, *Birth Control Laws*, 71.

22. Sheila Rothman, "Women's Clinics or Doctors' Offices: The Sheppard-Towner Act and the Promotion of Preventive Health Care," in *Social History and Social Policy*, ed. David J. Rothman and Stanton Wheeler (New York: Academic Press, 1981), 194.

23. Ibid., 158.

24. Dennett, "The Case for Birth Control," *Arbitrator*, n.d., box 13, MWD Papers. Dennett was identified as the secretary of the National Birth Control League in this article, so it must have been written before her resignation from the NBCL in March, 1919.

25. Dennett, *Birth Control Laws*, 92.

26. Ibid.

27. Chen, *The Sex Side of Life*, 143.

28. Dennett, letter of resignation from NBCL, March 5, 1919, box 15, MWD Papers.

29. Michael McGerr, "Political Style and Women's Power, 1830–1930," *Journal of American History* 77 (December 1990): 864–85.

30. On women's political power after suffrage, see McGerr, "Political Style and Women's Power"; Cott, *The Grounding of Modern Feminism*; Lemons, *The Woman Citizen*; Scharf and Jensen eds., *Decades of Discontent*.

31. It is important to note that, despite the CB's efforts, the three states that rejected Sheppard-Towner—Connecticut, Massachusetts, and Illinois—had large Catholic populations that continued to advance the notion that Sheppard-Towner was associated with birth control.

32. Sanger, "A Birth Strike to Avert World Famine," editorial in *BCR* 4, no.1 (January 1920), 1. In this editorial, she argued, "It is time for the women of the world—for each individual woman to accept her share of the problem. In this hour of crisis and peril, women alone can save the world."

33. Dennett, resignation from board of *Birth Control Review*, January 1920, box 16, MWD Papers.

34. Ibid.

35. Ibid.

36. T. H. Marshall, *Citizenship and Social Class* (New York: Cambridge University Press, 1950), quoted in Michel, *Children's Interests/Mothers' Rights*, 2.

37. One of the lessons reformers learned through their experience with the Sheppard-Towner Act was that self-interest and desire for control could motivate physicians as much as it could others in the professional sphere.

38. New York Academy of Medicine, Public Health Committee to Dennett, April 16, 1920, box 13, MWD Papers.

39. Dennett, "The Laws Against Contraceptive Knowledge," September 1921, box 15, MWD Papers.

40. Dennett to Putnam, September 9, 1919, box 30, ELP Papers.

41. Margaret Sanger, "Intelligence Tests for Legislators," *Birth Control Review* 7 (May 1923), 107.

42. Ibid.

43. *Birth Control Herald* 1 (January 12, 1923), 1.

44. Dennett, *Birth Control Laws*, 173.

45. Dennett, diaries and campaign reports, December 7, 1920, box 14, MWD Papers. This personal conflict of interest between Sheppard-Towner and the birth control bill is but a small reflection of a larger political conflict more fully explored in Robyn Rosen, "Federal Expansion, Fertility Control, and Physicians in the U.S.: The Politics of Maternal Welfare in the Interwar Years," *Journal of Women's History* 10, no. 3 (autumn 1998): 53–73.

46. Dennett, diaries and campaign reports, December 15, 1920, box 14, MWD Papers.

47. Dennett, *Birth Control Laws*, 95.

48. Dennett, "The Laws Against Contraceptive Knowledge," September 1921, box 15, MWD Papers.

49. Supplement to the *Birth Control Herald* 1 (May 15, 1923): Report of the Annual Meeting of the VPL, April 24, 1923.

50. *Birth Control Herald* 1 (March 8, 1923), 1.

51. Ibid.

52. Glases is quoted in Dennett, *Birth Control Laws*, 135, 136.

53. *Birth Control Herald* 1 (March 8, 1923), 1.

54. Ann Kennedy to Members of the VPL, n.d., box 19, MWD Papers.

55. Ibid.

56. Dennett to Senator Cummins, March 20, 1925, box 14, MWD Papers.

57. Ibid.

58. Ibid.

59. Ibid.

60. Ibid.

61. Bronson to Dennett, February 12, 1925, box 14, MWD Papers.

62. Bronson to Dennett, February 18, 1925, box 14, MWD Papers.

63. It was later reported that both groups refused to participate, November 1925, box 14, MWD Papers.

64. Minutes of Round Table Conference, April 6, 1926, box 15, MWD Papers.

65. Bronson to Dennett, September 10, 1925, box 14, MWD Papers.

66. Dennett to Bronson, September 18, 1925, box 14, MWD Papers.

67. Dennett, *Birth Control Laws*, 92, 266.

68. Myra P. Gallert, memo to VPL members, December 2, 1925, box 14, MWD Papers.

69. Dennett to Representative Vaile, January 30, 1926, box 17, MWD Papers.

70. Dennett, letter sent to various legislators praising a speech by President Coolidge, December 9, 1924, box 17, MWD Papers.

71. *Birth Control Review* 1 (February 1917), 3.

72. *Birth Control Herald* 1 (January 12, 1923), 4.

73. Sanger, "Editorial," *BCR* 5 (March 1921), 4.

74. McCann has a different interpretation of this split. She argues that Dennett's open bill "attempted to reestablish the free market in birth control that had existed

prior to the Comstock law's enactment. . . . Contraception was an entirely private matter; the government had no business interfering with individuals' free exercise of the private rights. Rhetoric in support of the doctors-only bill recognized the danger of capitalist market relations; it was the onus of these relations that justified the bill's restrictions" (70, 71). Here, McCann attributes Sanger's position not to expediency but solely to social welfare concerns, whereas I think it was a combination of both. Similarly, she oversimplifies Dennett's politics in her discussion of the free market. Dennett believed in free speech and the free flow of ideas, but this did not necessarily automatically translate into support for free market capitalism. I only agree with McCann to the extent that Dennett's formulation was clearly less sensitive than Sanger's to the issues of access and provision. McCann calls Dennett's bill "ideologically outdated" in its laissez-faire orientation, as opposed to the more up-to-date social welfare orientation of Sanger's bill. However, I would argue that, during the 1920s, as conservatives were in the White House, progressivism was in retreat, and maternalism as the foundation for social welfare was floundering, Dennett's bill was quite current and compatible with the decade.

75. Dennett's response to letters requesting birth control information is quoted in Chen, *The Sex Side of Life*, 215.

76. McCann, *Birth Control Politics in the U.S.*, 122, 123.

77. Ibid., 133.

78. Ibid.

79. Ibid.

80. Ibid. Italics mine.

81. Ibid.

82. Ibid.

83. Emma Goldman, "Observations and Comments," *Mother Earth* 10 (October 1915): 261, 262. When Goldman wrote this article, eugenic sterilization laws in the United States were in the process of being constitutionally challenged, and by 1918 all the state laws in existence were declared invalid. See Philip R. Reily, *The Surgical Solution: A History of Involuntary Sterilization in the United States* (Baltimore, Md.: Johns Hopkins University Press, 1991), 40.

84. Reily, *Surgical Solution*, 89, 121.

85. It was unclear whether Senator Cummins or Representative Vaile wrote this letter to Sonia Bronson, January 16, 1926, box 14, MWD Papers.

86. Dennett, *Who's Obscene?*, 10.

87. This conversion from Sanger's to Dennett's orientation was all but moot because, by 1936, the U.S. Supreme Court had ruled in *U.S. v. One Package* that birth control could be sent to physicians through the mail, causing legislative efforts to evaporate.

88. On the Dennett trial, see John M. Craig, "'The Sex Side of Life': The Obscenity Trial of Mary Ware Dennett," *Frontiers* 15, no. 3 (1995): 145–66; Constance Chen, *The Sex Side of Life*; and Leigh Ann Wheeler, *Rescuing Sex from Prudery and Prurience: Women's Politics and Anti-Obscenity Activism in the United States, 1910–1935* (Baltimore, Md.: Johns Hopkins University Press, forthcoming). While each provides important information (and, especially in the latter case, interesting analysis), none of these accounts of the trial considers its impact on Dennett's birth control activities.

89. Alan Reitman, ed., *The Pulse of Freedom: American Liberties 1920–1970s* (New York: W. W. Norton and Co., 1975), 57–59. Dennett's accusation against the DAR

reflects the growing rifts in the women's movement in the 1920s. The DAR was among the first women's groups to begin to disassociate itself from its more liberal and left-wing sisters during the post–World War I Red Scare. See Jensen, "All Pink Sisters" and Cott, *The Grounding of Modern Feminism.*

90. Dennett, letter to friends, February 20, 1929, box 24, MWD Papers.

91. Konikow to Dennett, April 29, 1929, box 25, MWD Papers.

92. Konikow to Dennett, July 3, 1929, box 25, MWD Papers.

93. Mary L. East to Dennett, April 1929, box 26, MWD Papers.

94. *Birth Control Review* 13 (June 1929), 148–51.

95. Dennett, *Who's Obscene?*, 183.

96. Reitman, *Pulse of Freedom*, 59.

97. A few years after the Dennett trial Ernst would argue the landmark case, *U.S. v. One Package.* For a more detailed account of the trial and its legal implications, see John M. Craig, "'The Sex Side of Life.'" See also Chen, *The Sex Side of Life*, chs. 16, 17, 18.

98. Dennett, *Who's Obscene?*, 195.

99. Craig, "'The Sex Side of Life'" and Chen, *Sex Side of Life*, chs. 16, 17, 18.

100. Dennett to Eleanor Jones, October 19, 1930, box 18, MWD Papers.

101. It seems more than coincidental that Putnam began to write about sex education and the dangers of censorship, and even began toying with the idea of birth control, in these years. In addition to arousing the support of outraged liberals, Dennett's calls for an end to government censorship appealed to a broader audience. Putnam, ever vigilant about the creeping intrusion of government in private life, also launched a critique of the Comstock Laws.

102. Dennett to Mary L. East, May 7, 1929, box 10, Planned Parenthood League of Massachusetts Papers (hereafter cited as PPLM Papers).

103. P. B. Huse to Dennett, October 1, 1929, box 18, MWD Papers.

104. Dennett to Gallert, October 3, 1929, box 20, MWD Papers.

105. Dennett to Gallert, February 9, 1930, box 20, MWD Papers.

106. Jones to Dennett, October 16, 1930, box 18, MWD Papers.

107. Dennett to Sanger, February 28,1931, box 22, MWD Papers.

108. Kate Crane Gartz to Sanger, March 28, 1931, box 23, MWD Papers.

109. Roger Baldwin to Dennett, December 10, 1934, box 18, MWD Papers.

110. Dennett to Baldwin, December 11, 1934, box 18, MWD Papers.

111. Ibid.

112. Baldwin to Dennett, December 13, 1934, box 18, MWD Papers.

113. Dennett, *Who's Obscene?*, 265.

114. Marguerite Benson to Dennett, March 16, 1936, box 18, MWD Papers.

115. Dennett to Marguerite Benson, March 18, 1936, box 18, MWD Papers.

116. Ibid.

117. Ibid.

118. Judge Augustus Hand, quoted in David M. Kennedy, *Birth Control in America: The Career of Margaret Sanger* (New Haven, Conn.: Yale University Press, 1970), 249.

119. Ibid, 249.

120. Ibid, 250.

121. Interesting parallels exist between Dennett's dissatisfaction with *U.S. v. One Package* and many feminists' disappointment with *Roe v. Wade.* In both cases, activists

worried that the decisions did not go far enough to firmly establish woman's right to control her body, but instead enhanced the power of physicians.

122. Ernst quoted in Chesler, *Woman of Valor,* 375.

123. Dennett to Edward Bruce, special advisor, Public Works of Art Project, Treasury Department, Washington, D.C., July 3, 1935, box 9, MWD Papers.

Notes to Chapter 4

1. Ames, diary entry, n.d., quoted in James Kenneally, *Blanche Ames and Woman Suffrage,* published lecture given at the Annual Meeting of the Friends of Borderland, Borderland State Park, Easton, Mass., 1992.

2. Kenneally, *Blanche Ames and Woman Suffrage,* 12–14, 23.

3. Dennett, *Birth Control Laws,* 10.

4. Dennett was responding to this need for clarification and comparison when she wrote *Birth Control Laws* in 1926. Here, she laid out her case against a state-by-state reform strategy that she considered inefficient and ineffective in the face of an overwhelming variety of obstacles.

5. Prescott Hall to BCLM, May 1917, box 38, PPLM Papers (Italics mine).

6. Blanche Ames to members of the Birth Control League, n.d., box 36, Ames Family Papers.

7. Anon., "Objects of the FWF," May 1919, box 25, PPLM Papers.

8. In her letter, East quotes Ames's criticisms and asks if she likes the revised objectives any better. May 5, 1919, box 36, Ames Family Papers.

9. Ames's independence from Sanger was surely forged from her experiences as a veteran of the embattled Massachusetts suffrage movement. For a brief account of the obstacles that Massachusetts suffragists faced, see Eleanor Flexner, *Century of Struggle: The Woman's Rights Movement in the United States* (Cambridge, Mass.: Harvard University Press, 1959), 230, 280, 281, 303, 306.

10. Advisory Board, BCLM, memorandum, July 29, 1919, box 38, Ames Family Papers. Dennett clearly shared this desire to not raise antagonism; she also wanted to disassociate from the radical implications and origins of the birth control movement. But in the same year the FWF was created, Dennett began her ambitious federal reform campaign in Washington, D.C., illustrating that her politics were not purely based on timidity, but, rather, on a sincere desire to advance the movement.

11. Advisory Board, BCLM, memo, July 29, 1919. McCann would argue that this appeal was doomed to fail because of the difference in sexual orientation between birth control reformers and welfare feminists. However, what interests me here is the lengths the FWF would go to in order to repackage their program into one that might fit with larger social welfare efforts during and after the war.

12. In 1916 the Children's Bureau published a study of maternal mortality. Meckel argues that, by the end of the second decade of the twentieth century, the two issues of infant and maternal mortality were inextricably linked in the minds of most reformers. However, Meckel does not address the role the birth control movement attempted to play in these campaigns. McCann argues that birth control must be seen in the context of other threads of activism on behalf of mothers and children in this period, but her emphasis is on the failure of birth controllers to convince welfare feminists to include birth control in their platform. McCann shows that, once rebuffed by

maternalists, Sangerists moved toward eugenics to popularize their cause. My study of Dennett and Ames shows options that existed to those who rejected eugenics but remained committed to the cause in the interwar years.

13. Mary L. East, "Conservation of Infant and Maternal Life," 1919, box 38, Ames Family Papers.

14. Vera P. Lane to Elizabeth Lowell Putnam, August 4, 1919, box 36, Ames Family Papers.

15. Dennett to Vera P. Lane, June 26, 1919, box 37, Ames Family Papers.

16. Dennett to Cerise Carmen Jack, June 4, 1919, box 37, Ames Family Papers.

17. Ibid.

18. Recall Konikow's letter to Dennett, in which she writes that, "The only energetic person in the crowd is Mrs. Oakes [Blanche] Ames." July 3, 1929, box 25, MWD Papers.

19. Lane to Dennett, September 30, 1919, box 26, Ames Family Papers.

20. The first issue of the *Birth Control Review* was published in 1917 and became the official organ of the ABCL in 1922. It served as an instrument of propaganda and as a way for local leagues to keep each other abreast of progress and obstacles encountered in their home states.

21. Secretary of Margaret Sanger to Lane, October 18, 1919, box 36, Ames Family Papers.

22. Ames, "Margaret Sanger's Influence," a paper written for the PPLM, 1958, box 42, Ames Family Papers.

23. Chesler, *Woman of Valor*, 226.

24. McCann provides an excellent chronology of events from 1916–1945 in *Birth Control Politics*, 209–18.

25. Scharf and Jensen argue that, during the interwar years, "The economic structure, the political institutions, and the social ideology all made it possible for individual women to achieve. The same conditions made it difficult for the women's movement to either maintain its strength or expand as an organized group committed to social change in opposition to the established order." Lois Scharf and Joan M. Jensen, eds., *Decades of Discontent: The Women's Movement, 1920–1940* (Boston: Northeastern University Press, 1987), 4.

26. See Reed, Kennedy, Gordon, McCann, Chesler. [au: James or Ruth Reed?]

27. James Reed, *From Private Vice to Public Virtue: The Birth Control Movement in American Society since 1830* (New York: Basic Books, 1978), 101. For more on the shift to a medical orientation and its political consequences, see Robyn Rosen, "Federal Expansion, Fertility Control, and Physicians in the U.S."

28. Ibid.

29. Annual Report of the BCLM, May 1, 1930, box 26, PPLM Papers.

30. Huthmacher, *Massachusetts People and Politics*, 70, 71.

31. Ibid., 68, 69.

32. C. R. Clapp to Ames, May 10, 1929, box 83, PPLM Papers.

33. Ibid.

34. East to members of the BCLM, November 1929, box 36, Ames Family Papers.

35. East, form letter, January 28, 1930, box 27, PPLM Papers.

36. Ibid.

37. Petitions, January 9, 1930, *Journal of the House of Representatives of the*

Commonwealth of Massachusetts (Boston: Wright and Potter Printing Co., Legislative Printers, 1930), 76.

38. East, Annual Report of the BCLM, May 1, 1930.

39. Ibid.

40. It is interesting to recall that, just as birth control activists in Massachusetts became increasingly committed to the doctors-only strategy, prominent members of the ABCL were beginning to embrace Dennett's perspective.

41. Petitions, *Journal of the Senate, Special Session, of the Commonwealth of Massachusetts, 1930–31,* January 7, 1931, 24.

42. Ames to Mrs. Hawkridge, October 29, 1930, box 36, PPLM Papers.

43. Ames, form letter, December 31, 1930, box 41, PPLM Papers.

44. Ibid.

45. Ibid.

46. East to Ames, January 26, 1931, box 36, PPLM Papers.

47. Ames, form letter, February 23, 1931, box 27, PPLM Papers.

48. Chesler, *Woman of Valor,* 318–24.

49. Linda Gordon, *Woman's Body, Woman's Right* (New York: Penguin, 1977), 269.

50. The quote from Himes's letter of resignation is found in Ames's letter to Himes, April 13, 1931, box 36, PPLM Papers.

51. Ames to Himes, April 13, 1931.

52. Ibid.

53. Ames, form letter, May 1931, box 27, PPLM Papers.

54. Murray F. Hall, legal opinion, February 5, 1932, box 83, PPLM Papers.

55. Ibid.

56. Ames, form letter, January 19, 1932, box 27, PPLM Papers.

57. Ames, form letter, 1931, box 27, PPLM Papers.

58. Ames, "Permission vs. Prohibition: The Rights of Physicians to Give Contraceptive Advice in Massachusetts and a Summary of Existing Legislation Throughout the U.S. Concerning Physicians and the Prevention of Conception," April 1932, box 42a, PPLM Papers.

59. Ibid.

60. Ames to Sanger, June 29, 1934, box 37, Ames Family Papers.

61. Ames, speech delivered before the Chicago Woman's City Club, n.d., box 32, PPLM Papers.

62. BCLM to Sanger, May 12, 1934, box 37, Ames Family Papers.

63. Ibid.

64. Ibid.

65. Sanger is quoted in the BCLM's responding letter, June 29, 1934, box 37, Ames Family Papers.

66. BCLM to Sanger, June 29, 1934, box 37, Ames Family Papers.

67. Ames to Mrs. Phillips, 1936, box 30, PPLM Papers.

68. Ibid.

69. The BCLM was still operating under the assumption that it could not advertise its clinics as "birth control clinics" under restrictive state statutes. The term "MHO" illustrates yet another euphemism used by the League to undercut the opposition.

70. Throughout the 1930s, the pages of the *BCR* are filled with references to "relief babies." Many contributors pointed to the amount of money spent (or, as some

said, wasted) on the unfit or unproductive elements of society. See Linda Gordon and Carole McCann for different but compatible interpretations of these trends in the movement.

71. Ames, Welfare Committee of the BCLM to female directors of women's work under the Civil Works Administration and other welfare committees, January 1934, box B-20, BCLM Papers, Schlesinger Library.

72. Ames, form letter, n.d., (1930–35), box 27, PPLM Papers.

73. Ibid.

74. Ibid.

75. Mary Irene Atkinson to Mrs. Tom Ragland, July 16, 1938, quoted in Kennedy, *Birth Control in America*, 261.

76. Ames, Welfare Committee of the BCLM to female directors of women's work under the Civil Works Administration and other welfare committees, January 1934. (Italics mine)

77. *Boston Transcript*, January 5, 1935, box 39, Ames Family Papers.

78. Ames to Executive Committee of the BCLM, January 8, 1935, box 39, Ames Family Papers.

79. Ames to Cannon, January 1935, box 39, Ames Family Papers.

80. Kennedy, *Birth Control In America*, 121.

81. Gordon, *Woman's Body, Woman's Right*, 284.

82. Anon., Pennsylvania Birth Control Federation, n.d., box 42a, PPLM Papers.

83. Ames to BCLM members, January 25, 1935, box 39, Ames Family Papers.

84. Ibid.

85. Ames, "Conflicting Views on Methods of Progress, Change of Constitution," n.d., box 39, Ames Family Papers.

86. Ibid.

87. Ames to Sanger, June 29, 1934, box 37, Ames Family Papers. (Italics mine)

88. Chesler argues that, by 1935 "the complexities of politics in Washington wore [Sanger] down," 356.

89. Ames to Mrs. Phillips, 1936, box 30, PPLM Papers.

90. Ibid.

91. For information on the ABCL in the mid-30s see McCann, *Birth Control Politics in the U.S.*, 178–180.

92. Kennedy, *Birth Control in America*, 213.

93. Anon., June 3, 1937, box 85, PPLM Papers.

94. Ibid.

95. BCLM, press release, quoted by Leslie D. Hawkridge, July 13, 1937, box 83, PPLM Papers.

96. BCLM, press release, October 15, 1937, box 83, PPLM Papers.

97. Dr. George Gilbert Smith to Members of the Massachusetts Medical Society, October 1937, box 27, PPLM Papers. Notes on the letter say that 5,101 letters were sent and the BCLM received 1,804 replies, with 1,790 signing in agreement of protest. Eight opposing letters were received, along with six noncommittal ones.

98. Ibid.

99. "Massachusetts Physicians and Birth Control," Editorial, *New England Journal of Medicine*, August 12, 1937, box 32, PPLM Papers.

100. Ibid.

101. *Commonwealth v. Gardner*, 15 N.E. 2d (1938), 372.

102. Ibid., 374.
103. Ibid., 374, 375.
104. Ibid., 375.
105. Ibid., 377.
106. BCLM, press release, May 26, 1938, box 83, PPLM Papers.
107. Ibid.
108. BCLM press release, May 27, 1938, box 83, PPLM Papers.
109. BCLM, conference report, June 1938, box 64, PPLM Papers.
110. Anon., memorandum, November 1938, box 30, PPLM Papers.
111. BCLM, news release, January 17, 1939, box 32b, PPLM Papers.
112. Editorial, *New England Journal of Medicine* 220, no.1 (January 5, 1939), 37–38.
113. BCLM, form letter, March 1939, box 27, PPLM Papers.
114. Ibid.
115. Ibid.
116. BCLM, executive board correspondence, announcement of new name and move to Newbury Street, April 4, 1939, box 26, PPLM Papers.
117. Commonwealth vs. Corbett, 307 Mass. 7 (1940), 8.
118. Ibid., 14.
119. Helena M. Wall, "Feminism and the New England Hospital, 1949–1961," 435.
120. Ibid., 438.

Notes to Epilogue

1. Kathryn Kish Sklar, *Florence Kelley and the Nation's Work*, vol. 1 (New Haven, Conn.: Yale University Press, 1995), xv, xvi.

Bibliography

Manuscript Collections

Ames, Blanche A. Papers. Schlesinger Library, Radcliffe College, Cambridge, Mass.

Ames Family Papers. Sophia Smith Collection, Smith College, Northampton, Mass.

Birth Control League of Massachusetts Papers, Schlesinger Library, Cambridge, Mass.

Brown, Dorothy Kirchwey. Papers. Schlesinger Library, Radcliffe College, Cambridge, Mass.

Bureau of Social Hygiene. Archives, 1911–1940. Rockefeller Archives Center, North Tarrytown, N.Y.

Dennett, Mary Ware. Papers. Schlesinger Library, Radcliffe College, Cambridge, Mass.

Dummer, Ethel Sturges. Papers. Schlesinger Library, Radcliffe College, Cambridge, Mass.

Laura Spelman Rockefeller Memorial. Archives, 1918–1949. Rockefeller Archives Center, North Tarrytown, N.Y.

Planned Parenthood League of Massachusetts Papers. Sophia Smith Collection, Smith College, Northampton, Mass.

Putnam, Elizabeth Lowell. Papers. Schlesinger Library, Radcliffe College, Cambridge, Mass.

Rockefeller Family Archives. Office of Messrs. Rockefeller. Medical Interests, 1894–1962. Rockefeller Archives Center, North Tarrytown, N.Y.

Russell Sage Foundation. Records, 1885–1982. Rockefeller Archives Center, North Tarrytown, N.Y.

Sanger, Margaret. Papers. Sophia Smith Collection, Smith College, Northampton, Mass.

Stöcker, Helene. Papers. Swarthmore College Peace Collection, Swarthmore College, Swarthmore, Pa.

United States Children's Bureau. Central File Records, 1914–1968. National Archives, Washington, D.C.

Newspapers and Journals

Birth Control Herald
Birth Control Review
Boston Herald
The Forerunner
Journal of the American Medical Association
Mother Earth
New England Journal of Medicine
The Survey

Books, Articles, and Unpublished Studies

Abramovitz, Mimi. *Regulating the Lives of Women: Social Welfare Policy from Colonial Times to the Present.* Boston: South End Press, 1988.

Addams, Jane. *My Friend, Julia Lathrop.* New York: Macmillan, 1935; reprint, New York: Arno Press, 1974.

Allen, Ann Taylor. *Feminism and Motherhood in Germany 1800–1914.* New Brunswick, N.J.: Rutgers University Press, 1991.

———."German Radical Feminism and Eugenics, 1900–1918." *German Studies Review* 11 (February 1988): 31–56.

———. "Mothers of the New Generation: Adele Schreiber, Helene Stoecker, and the Evolution of a German Idea of Motherhood." *Signs* 10 (spring 1985): 418–38.

Alonso, Harriet. *Peace as a Women's Issue: A History of the U.S. Movement for World Peace and Women's Rights.* Syracuse, N.Y.: Syracuse University Press, 1993.

———. *The Women's Peace Union and the Outlawry of War, 1921–1942.* Knoxville: University of Tennessee Press, 1989.

Anthony, Katharine. *Feminism in Germany and Scandinavia.* New York: Henry Holt, 1915.

———. *Mothers Who Must Earn.* New York: Trow Press, 1914.

———, ed. *The Endowment of Motherhood.* New York: B. W. Huebsch, Inc., 1920.

Antler, Joyce, and Daniel M. Fox. "The Movement Toward Safe Maternity: Physician Accountability in New York City, 1915–1940." In *Sickness and Health in America,* edited by Judith Walzer Leavitt and Ronald L. Numbers. Madison: University of Wisconsin Press, 1985.

Apple, Rima D. *Mothers and Medicine: A Social History of Infant Feeding, 1880–1950.* Madison: University of Wisconsin Press, 1987.

Baker, Paula. "The Domestication of Politics: Women and American Political Society, 1780–1920." *American Historical Review* 89 (June 1984): 620–47.

Baker, S. Josephine. *Fighting for Life.* New York: Macmillan, 1939; reprint, New York: Arno Press, 1974.

Bederman, Gail. *Manliness and Civilization: A Cultural History of Gender and Race in the United States, 1880–191.* Chicago: University of Chicago Press, 1995.

Berkowitz, Edward D. *America's Welfare State: From Roosevelt to Reagan.* Baltimore, Md.: Johns Hopkins Press, 1991.

Blair, Karen. *The Clubwoman as Feminist: True Womanhood Redefined, 1868–1914.* New York: Holmes & Meier Publishers, 1980.

Bordin, Ruth. *Women and Temperance: The Quest for Power and Liberty, 1873–1900.* Philadelphia: University of Pennsylvania Press, 1981.

Boris, Eileen. "The Power of Motherhood: Black and White Activist Women Redefine the 'Political.'" In *Mothers of a New World,* edited by Seth Koven and Sonya Michel, 213–45. New York: Routledge, 1993.

———. "Reconstructing the Family: Women, Progressive Reform, and the Problem of Social Control." In *Gender, Race, Class and Reform in the Progressive Era,* edited by Noralee Frankel and Nancy S. Dye, 73–86. Lexington: University Press of Kentucky, 1991.

Brandt, Allan M. *No Magic Bullet: A Social History of Venereal Disease in the United States Since 1880.* New York: Oxford University Press, 1987.

Bremner, Robert H. *From the Depths: The Discovery of Poverty in the United States.* New York: New York University Press, 1956.

Bridenthal, Renate, et al., *When Biology Became Destiny: Women in Weimar and Nazi Germany.* New York: Monthly Review Press, 1984.

Buhle, Mari Jo. *Women and American Socialism, 1870–1920.* Urbana: University of Illinois Press, 1981.

Chen, Constance M. *The Sex Side of Life: Mary Ware Dennett's Pioneering Battle for Birth Control and Sex Education.* New York: New York Press, 1996.

Chepaitis, Joseph Benedict. "The First Federal Social Welfare Measure: The Sheppard-Towner Maternity and Infancy Act, 1918–1932." Ph.D. diss., Georgetown University, 1968.

Chesler, Ellen. *Woman of Valor: Margaret Sanger and the Birth Control Movement in America.* New York: Simon and Schuster, 1992.

Cook, Blanche Weisen. *Crystal Eastman on Women and Revolution.* New York: Oxford, 1979.

———. "Female Support Networks and Political Activism: Lillian Wald, Crystal Eastman, Emma Goldman." In *A Heritage of Her Own: Toward a New Social History of American Women,* edited by Nancy F. Cott and Elizabeth H. Pleck, 412–44. New York: Simon and Schuster, 1979.

Costin, Leila B. *Two Sisters for Social Justice: A Biography of Grace and Edith Abbott.* Urbana: University of Illinois Press, 1983.

Cott, Nancy F. *The Grounding of Modern Feminism.* New Haven, Conn.: Yale University Press, 1987.

———. "What's In a Name? The Limits of 'Social Feminism'; or, Expanding the Vocabulary of Women's History." *Journal of American History* 76 (December 1989): 809–29.

Covotsos, Louis J. "Child Welfare and Social Progress: A History of the United States Children's Bureau, 1912–35." Ph.D. diss., University of Chicago, 1976.

Craig, John M. "'The Sex Side of Life': The Obscenity Trial of Mary Ware Dennett." *Frontiers* 15, no. 3 (1995): 145–66.

Crocker, Ruth Hutchinson. *Social Work and Social Order.* Urbana: University of Illinois Press, 1992.

Curry, Lynne. *Modern Mothers in the Heartland: Gender, Health and Progress in Illinois, 1900–1930.* Columbus: Ohio State University Press, 1999.

Davis, Allen F. *Spearheads for Reform: The Social Settlements and the Progressive Movement, 1890–1914.* New Brunswick, N.J.: Rutgers University Press, 1984.

Deegan, Mary Jo. *Jane Addams and the Men of the Chicago School, 1892–1918.* New Brunswick, N.J.: Transaction Books, 1990, c1988.

Degen, Marie Louise. *The History of the Woman's Peace Party.* Baltimore, Md.: Johns Hopkins University Press, 1939.

D'Emilio, John, and Estelle Freedman. *Intimate Matters: A History of Sexuality in America.* New York: Harper and Row, 1988.

Dennett, Mary Ware. *Birth Control Laws: Shall We Keep Them, Change Them, or Abolish Them?* New York: Grafton Press, 1936.

————. *Who's Obscene?* New York: Vanguard Press, 1930.

Donohue, William A. *The Politics of the ACLU.* New Brunswick, N.J.: Transaction Books, 1985.

Douglas, Emily Taft. *Margaret Sanger: Pioneer of the Future.* New York: Holt, Rinehart, and Winston, 1970.

Dumenil, Lynn. "'The Insatiable Maw of Bureaucracy': Antistatism and Education Reform in the 1920s." *Journal of American History* 77 (September 1990): 499–524.

Dummer, Ethel Sturges. *Why I Think So: The Autobiography an Hypothesis.* Chicago: Clarke-McElroy Publishing Co., 1937.

Early, Frances. "Feminism, Peace, and Civil Liberties: Women's Role in the Origins of the World War I Civil Liberties Movement." *Women's Studies* 18 (1990): 95–115.

Epstein, Barbara Leslie. "Family, Sexual Morality, and Popular Movements in Turn-of-the-Century America." In *Powers of Desire: The Politics of Sexuality,* edited by Ann Snitow et al., 117–30. New York: Monthly Review Press, 1983.

————. *The Politics of Domesticity: Women, Evangelism, and Temperance in Nineteenth-Century America.* Middletown, Conn.: Wesleyan University Press, 1981.

Evans, Richard. *The Feminist Movement in Germany, 1984–1933.* London: Sage Publications, 1976.

Farrell, John C. *Beloved Lady: A History of Jane Addams' Ideas on Peace and Reform.* Baltimore, Md.: Johns Hopkins University Press, 1967.

Fee, Elizabeth, and Barbara Greene. "Science and Social Reform: Women and Public Health." *Journal of Public Health Policy* 10 (1989): 161–77.

Fitzpatrick, Ellen. *Endless Crusade: Women Social Scientists and Progressive Reform.* New York: Oxford University Press, 1990.

Flanagan, Maureen A. "Gender and Urban Political Reform: The City Club and the Woman's City Club of Chicago in the Progressive Era." *American Historical Review* 95 (October 1990): 1032–50.

Flexner, Eleanor. *Century of Struggle: The Woman's Rights Movement in the United States.* Cambridge, Mass.: Harvard University Press, 1959.

Fox-Genovese, Elizabeth. *Feminism without Illusions: A Critique of Individualism.* Chapel Hill: University of North Carolina Press, 1991.

Freedman, Estelle. *Maternal Justice: Miriam Van Waters and the Female Reform Tradition.* Chicago: University of Chicago Press, 1996.

Friend, Ernst. *Illegitimacy Laws of the United States and Certain Foreign Countries.* U.S. Children's Bureau Publication No. 42, Legal Series No. 2. Washington, D.C.: Government Printing Office, 1919.

Fryer. Peter. *The Birth Controllers.* New York: Stein & Day, 1965.

Ginzberg, Lori. *Women and the Work of Benevolence: Morality, Politics and Class in the Nineteenth Century United States.* New Haven, Conn.: Yale University Press, 1990.

Glover, Katherine, and Evelyn Dewey. *Children of the New Day.* New York: D. Appleton, 1934.

Goodwin, Joanne L. "An Experiment in Paid Motherhood: The Implementation of Mothers' Pensions in Early Twentieth Century Chicago." *Gender & History* 4 (autumn 1992): 323–42.

———. *Gender and the Politics of Welfare Reform.* Chicago: University of Chicago Press, 1997.

Gordon, Felicia. "Reproductive Rights: The Early Twentieth Century European Debate." *Gender & History* 4 (autumn 1992): 387–99.

Gordon, Linda. "Black and White Visions of Welfare: Women's Welfare Activism, 1890–1945." *Journal of American History* 78 (September 1991): 559–90.

———. *Pitied but Not Entitled: Single Mothers and the History of Welfare, 1890–1935.* New York: Free Press, 1994.

———. "Social Insurance and Public Assistance: The Influence of Gender in Welfare Thought in the United States, 1890–1935." *American Historical Review* 97 (February 1992): 19–54.

———. "What Does Welfare Regulate?" *Social Research* 55 (winter 1988): 609–30.

———. *Woman's Body, Woman's Right.* New York: Penguin, 1977.

———. *Women, the State, and Welfare.* Madison: University of Wisconsin Press, 1990.

Gray, Madeline. *Margaret Sanger: A Biography of the Champion of Birth Control.* New York: Richard Marek Publishers, 1979.

Grossman, Atina. "The New Woman and the Rationalization of Sexuality in Weimar Germany." In *Powers of Desire: The Politics of Sexuality,* edited by Ann Snitow et al., 153–76. New York: Monthly Review Press, 1983.

———. "The New Woman, the New Family and the Rationalization of Sexuality: The Sex Reform Movement in Germany 1928 to 1933." Ph.D. diss., Rutgers University, 1984.

———. *Reforming Sex: The German Movement for Birth Control and Abortion Reform, 1920–1950.* New York: Oxford University Press, 1995.

Hackett, Amy. "Helene Stoecker: Left-Wing Intellectual and Sex Reformer." In *When Biology Became Destiny: Women in Weimar and Nazi Germany,* edited by Bridenthal et al., 109–30. New York: Monthly Review Press, 1984.

———. "The Politics of Feminism in Wilhelmine Germany 1880–1918." Ph.D. diss., Columbia University, 1976.

Haskell, Thomas. *The Emergence of Professional Social Science.* Urbana: University of Illinois Press, 1977.

Healy, William. *Harvey Humphrey Baker: Upbuilder of the Juvenile Court.* Boston: Judge Baker Foundation Publications, 1920.

———. *The Individual Delinquent.* Boston: Little, Brown, 1915.

Healy, William, and Augusta F. Bronner. *Delinquents and Criminals: Their Making and Unmaking.* New York: MacMillan, 1926.

Hirshfield, Daniel S. *The Lost Reform: The Campaign for Compulsory Health Insurance from 1932 to 1943.* Cambridge, Mass.: Harvard University Press, 1970.

Hobson, Barbara Meil. *Uneasy Virtue: The Politics of Prostitution and the American Reform Tradition.* New York: Basic Books, 1987.

Hoffert, Sylvia D. *Private Matters: American Attitudes Toward Childbearing and Infant Nurture in the Urban North, 1800–1860.* Urbana: University of Illinois Press, 1989.

Huthmacher, Joseph. *Massachusetts People and Politics, 1919–1933.* New York: Athenueum,1969.

Jensen, Joan. "All Pink Sisters: The War Department and the Feminist Movement in the 1920s." In *Decades of Discontent: The Women's Movement 1920–1940,* edited by Lois Scharf and Joan Jensen, 199–222. Boston: Northeastern University Press, 1987.

Jerome, Jane. *Women Against Women.* Brooklyn, N.Y.: Carlson, 1994.

Katz, Michael B. *In the Shadow of the Poorhouse: A Social History of Welfare in America.* New York: Basic Books, 1986.

Kenneally, James. *Blanche Ames and Woman Suffrage.* Published lecture given at the Annual Meeting of the Friends of Borderland, Borderland State Park, Easton, Mass., 1992.

Kennedy, David M. *Birth Control in America: The Career of Margaret Sanger.* New Haven, Conn.: Yale University Press, 1970.

Kessler-Harris, Alice. *Out to Work: A History of Wage-Earning Women in the United States.* New York: Oxford University Press, 1982.

Key, Ellen. *The Century of the Child.* New York: Putnam, 1909.

———. *The Renaissance of Motherhood.* New York, 1914.

Koven, Seth, and Sonya Michel. "Womanly Duties: Maternalist Politics and the Origins of the Welfare State in France, Germany, Great Britain, and the United States." *American Historical Review* 95 (October 1990): 1076–1108.

———, eds. *Mothers of a New World: Maternalist Politics and the Origins of Welfare States.* New York: Routledge, 1993.

Kraditor, Aileen S. *The Ideas of the Woman Suffrage Movement, 1890–1920.* New York: W. W. Norton, 1981.

Kunzel, Regina K. *Fallen Women, Problem Girls: Unmarried Mothers and the Professionalization of Social Work, 1890–1945.* New Haven, Conn.: Yale University Press, 1993.

Ladd-Taylor, Molly. "Hull House Goes to Washington: Women and the Children's Bureau." In *Gender, Race, Class and Reform in the Progressive Era,* edited by Noralee Frankel and Nancy S. Dye, 110–26. Lexington: University Press of Kentucky, 1991.

———. *Mother-Work: Women, Child Welfare, and the State, 1890–1930.* Urbana: University of Illinois Press, 1994.

———. "'My Work Came Out of Agony and Grief': Mothers and the Making of the Sheppard-Towner Act." In *Mothers of a New World,* edited by Seth Koven and Sonya Michel, 321–42. New York: Routledge, 1993.

———. *Raising a Baby the Government Way: Mothers' Letters to the Children's Bureau, 1915–32.* New Brunswick, N.J.: Rutgers University Press, 1986.

———. "Voluntary Organizations, State Activity and Policies Toward Mothers: The Sheppard-Towner Act." Unpublished paper presented at the Harvard Conference on Gender and the Welfare State, Cambridge, Mass. February, 1988.

Lader, Lawrence. *The Margaret Sanger Story and the Fight for Birth Control.* New York: Doubleday, 1955.

Lamson, Peggy. *Roger Baldwin: Founder of the ACLU.* Boston: Houghton Mifflin Co., 1976.

Leavitt, Judith Walzer. *Brought to Bed: Childbearing in America.* New York: Oxford University Press, 1986.

———. *The Healthiest City: Milwaukee and the Politics of Health Reform.* Princeton, N.J.: Princeton University Press, 1982.

Leff, Mark H. "Consensus for Reform: The Mothers' Pension Movement in the Progressive Era." In *Compassion and Responsibility: Readings in the History of Social Welfare Policy in the United States,* edited by Frank R. Breul and Steven J. Diner, 244–64. Chicago: University of Chicago Press, 1980.

Lemons, J. Stanley. *The Woman Citizen: Social Feminism in the 1920s.* Urbana: University of Illinois Press, 1975.

Lindenmeyer, Kriste. *"A Right to Childhood": The U.S. Children's Bureau and Child Welfare, 1912–46.* Urbana: University of Illinois Press, 1997.

Lunardini, Christine A. *From Equal Suffrage to Equal Rights: Alice Paul and the National Women's Party, 1910–1928.* New York: New York University Press, 1986.

Lundberg, Emma O. and Katherine Lenroot. *Illegitimacy as a Child Welfare Problem,* Pt. I: "A Brief Treatment of the Prevalence and Significance of Birth Out of Wedlock, the Child's Status, and the State's Responsibility for Care and Protection." U.S. Children's Bureau Publication No. 66. Washington, D.C.: Government Printing Office, 1920.

McCann, Carole R. *Birth Control Politics in the U.S., 1916–45.* Ithaca, N.Y.: Cornell University Press, 1994.

McCarthy, Kathleen. *Noblesse Oblige: Charity and Cultural Philanthropy in Chicago, 1849–1929.* Chicago: University of Chicago Press, 1982.

McGerr, Michael. "Political Style and Women's Power, 1830–1930." *Journal of American History* 77 (December 1990): 864–85.

McKeany, Maurine. *The Absent Father and Public Policy in the Program of Aid to Dependent Children.* University of California Publications in Social Welfare, Vol. 1. Edited by Ernest Greenwood, H. E. Jones, Davis McEntire. Berkeley: University of California Press, 1960.

Meckel, Richard A. *Save the Babies: American Public Health Reform and the Prevention of Infant Mortality, 1850–1929.* Baltimore, Md.: Johns Hopkins University Press, 1990.

Michel, Sonya. *Children's Interests/Mothers' Rights: The Shaping of America's Child Care Policy.* New Haven, Conn.: Yale University Press, 1999.

———. "From Civic Usefulness to Federal Maternalism: Social Feminism and the Rise of the American Welfare State," presented at the Seventh Berkshire Conference on the History of Women, Wellesley College, 1987.

———. "The Limits of Maternalism: Policies toward American Wage-Earning Mothers during the Progressive Era." In *Mothers of a New World,* edited by Seth Koven and Sonya Michel, 277–320. New York: Routledge, 1993.

Michel, Sonya, and Robyn L. Rosen. "The Paradox of Maternalism: Elizabeth Lowell Putnam and the Welfare State." *Gender and History* (fall 1992): 364–86.

Mink, Gwendolyn. "The Lady and the Tramp: Gender, Race, and the Origins of the American Welfare State." In *Women, the State, and Welfare,* edited by Linda Gordon, 92–121. Madison: University of Wisconsin Press, 1990.

———. *The Wages of Motherhood: Inequality in the Welfare State, 1917–1942.* Ithaca, N.Y.: Cornell University Press, 1995.

Muncy, Robyn. *Creating a Female Dominion in American Reform, 1890–1935.* New York: Oxford University Press, 1991.

Nelson, Barbara. "The Origins of the Two-Channel Welfare State: Workmen's

Compensation and Mothers' Aid." In *Women, the State, and Welfare,* edited by Linda Gordon, 123–51. Madison: University of Wisconsin Press, 1990.

Norwegian Laws Concerning Illegitimate Children. Washington, D.C.: Children's Bureau Publication, Legal Series no. 1, Bureau Publication no. 31, 1918.

Odem, Mary. *Delinquent Daughters: Protecting and Policing Adolescent Female Sexuality in the United States, 1885–1920.* Chapel Hill: University of North Carolina Press, 1995.

Offen, Karen. "Depopulation, Nationalism, and Feminism in Fin-de-Siècle France." *American Historical Review* 89 (1984): 654.

———. "Defining Feminism: A Comparative Historical Approach." *Signs* 14 (1988): 119–57.

O'Neill, William. *Everyone Was Brave: A History of Feminism in America.* New York: Quadrangle, 1971.

Pivan, Frances Fox, and Richard A. Cloward. *Regulating the Poor: The Functions of Public Welfare.* New York: Pantheon, 1971.

Pivar, David. *Purity and Hygiene: Women, Prostitution and the "American Plan," 1900–1930.* Westport, Conn.: Greenwood Press, 2002.

Platt, Anthony. *The Child Savers: The Invention of Delinquency.* Chicago: University of Chicago Press, 1969.

Platt, Jennifer. "Acting as a Switchboard." *The American Sociologist* (fall 1992): 23–36.

Puttee, Dorothy Frances, and Mary Ruth Colby. *The Illegitimate Child in Illinois.* Publication of the University of Chicago Social Service Monographs, edited by Sonia P. Breckinridge. Chicago: University of Chicago Press, 1937.

Reed, James. *From Private Vice to Public Virtue: The Birth Control Movement in American Society since 1830.* New York: Basic Books, 1978.

Reed, Ruth. *The Illegitimate Family in New York City: Its Treatment by Social and Health Agencies.* Studies of the Research Bureau of the Welfare Council of New York City, No. 11. New York: Columbia University Press, 1934.

Register, Cheri, "Motherhood at Center: Ellen Key's Social Vision." *Women's Studies International Forum* 5 (1982): 599–610.

Reily, Philip R. *The Surgical Solution: A History of Involuntary Sterilization in the United States.* Baltimore, Md.: Johns Hopkins University Press, 1991.

Reitman, Alan, ed. *The Pulse of Freedom: American Liberties 1920–1970s.* New York: W. W. Norton and Co., 1975.

Reynolds, Moira Davison. *Women Advocates of Reproductive Rights: Eleven Who Led the Struggle in the United States and Great Britain.* Jefferson, N.C.: McFarland & Company, 1994.

Rosen, George. *Preventive Medicine in the United State, 1900–1975.* New York: Science History Publications, 1975.

Rosen, Robyn. "Federal Expansion, Fertility Control, and Physicians in the U.S.: The Politics of Maternal Welfare in the Interwar Years." *Journal of Women's History* 10, no. 3 (autumn 1998): 53–73.

Rosen, Ruth. *The Lost Sisterhood: Prostitution in America 1900–1918.* Baltimore, Md.: Johns Hopkins University Press, 1981.

Rosenberg, Charles. *The Care of Strangers: The Rise of the American Hospital System.* New York: Basic Books, 1987.

Rosenberg, Rosalind. *Beyond Separate Spheres: Intellectual Roots of Modern Feminism.* New Haven, Conn.: Yale University Press, 1982.

Rosenkrantz, Barbara Gutmann. *Public Health and the State: Changing Views in Massachusetts, 1842–1936.* Cambridge, Mass.: Harvard University Press, 1972.

Rossiter, Margaret W. *Women Scientists in America.* Baltimore, Md.: Johns Hopkins University Press, 1982.

Rothman, David. *Conscience and Convenience: The Asylum and Its Alternatives in Progressive America.* Boston: Little, Brown, 1980.

Rothman, Sheila M. *Woman's Proper Place: A History of Changing Ideals and Practices, 1870 to the Present.* New York: Basic Books, 1978.

———. "Women's Clinics or Doctors' Offices: The Sheppard-Towner Act and the Promotion of Preventive Health Care." In *Social History and Social Policy,* edited by David J. Rothman and Stanton Wheeler. New York: Academic Press, 1981.

Ryan, Mary P. *Women in Public: From Banners to Ballots.* Baltimore, Md.: Johns Hopkins University Press, 1990.

Ryerson, Ellen. *Best Laid Plans: America's Juvenile Court Experiment.* New York: Hill & Wang, 1978.

Sanger, Margaret. *Margaret Sanger: An Autobiography.* 1938; reprint, New York: Dover Publications, Inc., 1971.

———. *Woman and the New Race.* New York: Brentanos, 1920.

Sapiro, Virginia. "The Gender Basis of American Social Policy." In *Women, the State, and Welfare,* edited by Linda Gordon, 36–54. Madison: University of Wisconsin Press, 1990.

Sarvasy, Wendy. "Beyond the Difference versus Equality Policy Debate: Postsuffrage Feminism, Citizenship, and the Quest for a Feminist Welfare State." *Signs* 17 (winter 1992): 329–62.

Scharf, Lois, and Joan M. Jensen, eds. *Decades of Discontent: The Women's Movement, 1920–1940.* Boston: Northeastern University Press, 1987.

Schlesinger, Edward R. "The Sheppard-Towner Era: A Prototype Case Study in Federal-State Relations." *American Journal of Public Health* 57, no. 6 (June 1967): 1034–41.

Schlossman, Steven L. *Love and the American Delinquent: The Theory and Practice of "Progressive" Juvenile Justice.* Chicago, University of Chicago Press, 1970.

Schneider, Eric C. *In the Web of Class: Delinquents and Reformers in Boston, 1810s–1930s.* New York: New York University Press, 1992.

Schwarz, Judith. *Radical Feminists of Heterodoxy: Greenwich Village 1912–40.* Lebanon, N.H.: New Victoria Press, 1982.

Sherman, Richard B. "Foss of Massachusetts: Demagogue or Progressive." *Mid-America* 43, no. 2 (April 1961): 75–94.

Silverberg, Helene, ed. *Gender and American Social Science: The Formative Years.* Princeton, N.J.: Princeton University Press, 1998.

Sklar, Kathryn Kish. "'Brain Work for Women': Women, Social Science, and the American Welfare State in the Progressive Era." Paper presented at the Eighth Berkshire Conference in Women's History, Douglass College, New Brunswick, N.J., June 1990.

———. *Florence Kelley and the Nation's Work.* New Haven, Conn.: Yale University Press, 1995.

———. "The Historical Foundations of Woman's Power in the creation of the American Welfare State." In *Mothers of a New World,* edited by Seth Koven and Sonya Michel, 43–92. New York: Routledge, 1993.

————. "Hull House in the 1890s: A Community of Women Reformers." *Signs* 10 (summer 1985): 658–77.

Skocpol, Theda. *Protecting Soldiers and Mothers: The Political Origins of Social Policy in the United States.* Cambridge, Mass.: Harvard University Press, 1992.

Smith, Susan L. *Sick and Tired of Being Sick and Tired: Black Women's Health Activism in America, 1890–1950.* Philadelphia: University of Pennsylvania Press, 1995.

Smith-Rosenberg, Carroll. *Disorderly Conduct: Visions of Gender in Victorian America.* New York: Oxford University Press, 1985.

Standards of Legal Protection for Children Born Out of Wedlock: A Report of Regional Conferences. Bureau Publication no. 77. Washington, D.C.: Government Printing Office, 1921.

Starr, Paul. *The Social Transformation of American Medicine: The Rise of a Sovereign Profession and the Making of a Vast Industry.* New York: Basic Books, 1982.

Stearns, Harold E., ed. *Civilization in the United States.* New York: Harcourt, 1922.

Thomas, William I. *The Unadjusted Girl With Cases and Standpoint for Behavior Analysis.* Boston: Little, Brown, 1923.

Tiffin, Susan. *In Whose Best Interest? Child Welfare Reform in the Progressive Era.* Westport, Conn.: Greenwood Press, 1982.

Tobey, James A. *The National Government and Public Health.* Baltimore, Md.: Johns Hopkins Press, 1926; reprint, New York: Arno Press, 1978.

Tomes, Nancy. *The Gospel of Germs: Men, Women and the Microbe in American Life.* Cambridge, Mass.: Harvard University Press, 1998.

Trattner, Walter I., ed. *From Poor Law to Welfare State: A History of Social Welfare in America.* New York: Free Press, 1984.

————. *Social Welfare or Social Control? Some Historical Reflections on Regulating the Poor.* Knoxville: University of Tennessee Press, 1983.

Trimberger, Ellen Kay. "Feminism, Men and Modern Love: Greenwich Village, 1900–1925." In *Powers of Desire: The Politics of Sexuality,* edited by Ann Snitow et al., 131–52. New York: Monthly Review Press, 1983.

Van Waters, Miriam. *Parents on Probation.* New York: New Republic, Inc., 1927; reprint, New York: Garland Publishing, 1987.

Veysey, Lawrence. *Emergence of the American University.* Chicago: University of Chicago Press, 1965.

Wall, Helena M. "Feminism and the New England Hospital, 1949–1961." *American Quarterly* 32 (1980): 430–45.

Wertz, Richard W., and Dorothy C. Wertz, *Lying In: A History of Childbirth in America.* New York: Schocken, 1979.

Wexler, Alice. *Emma Goldman in America.* Boston: Beacon Press, 1984.

Wheeler, Lee Ann. *Rescuing Sex from Prudery and Prurience: Women's Politics and Anti-Obscenity Activism in the United States, 1910–1935.* Baltimore, Md.: Johns Hopkins University Press, forthcoming.

Witte, Edwin E. *The Development of the Social Security Act.* Madison: University of Wisconsin Press, 1962.

Zimmerman, Joan G. "The Jurisprudence of Equality: The First Women's Minimum Wage, the First Equal Rights Amendment, and Adkins v. Children's Hospital, 1905–23." *Journal of American History* 78 (June 1991): 188–225.

Index